Advance Praise for *The Bitter Prescription*

"Dr. Stagg delivers a new framework of how we should eat as we age, so we can get rid of belly fat, improve our metabolism and digestive health, while also addressing the bitter emotions that age us prematurely—the complete package!"

—JJ Virgin, CNS, New York Times Bestselling Author
of The Virgin Diet

"Developing disease and losing function with aging is common—but is neither normal, nor inevitable. Follow Dr. Stagg's great, easily understood, and followed advice and get off the relentless disease train."

—Joseph Pizzorno, ND, Coauthor of the Multimillion-Copy Bestseller The
Encyclopedia of Natural Medicine

"In The Bitter Prescription, author Dr. Jennifer Stagg clearly draws on her backgrounds in biochemistry, nutrition, and naturopathic medicine to wonderfully weave a guide to living longer and living better. All of the most important elements are there, including prioritizing the quality and composition of the food that we eat, the regenerative powers of proper sleep, the importance of the kind of inner dialogue and thoughts that permeate our brains, and the importance of social networks. This is no fad diet book, but instead a comprehensive sensible lifestyle road map to adding years to life, and life to years."

—Dr. David Brady, Author of The Fibro Fix

"The Bitter Prescription is built on the scientific research and traditional aspects of how taste primes our body's response for health. This is such a fascinating guide that brings together not just the culmination of what you need to know from the research in this emerging area, but also the emotional-mental aspects of how we might manifest bitter in the psyche. Truly, a mind-body guide to living with food bitters and having less bitterness in one's life. A must read!"

—Deanna Minich, PhD, IFMCP, CNS, Author
of Whole Detox and The Rainbow Diet

"The Bitter Prescription is just what the doctor ordered as the bitter truth of aging hits us. From digestion and the fascinating science of bitter foods to advice on exercise, stress, and hormones, Dr. Stagg creates a timely and easy-to-follow guide that is sweet news."

—Robert Bonakdar MD FAAFP FACN, Director of Pain Management,
Scripps Center for Integrative Medicine

Also by Dr. Jennifer Stagg

Unzip Your Genes: 5 Choices to Reveal a Radically Radiant You

The *Bitter Prescription*

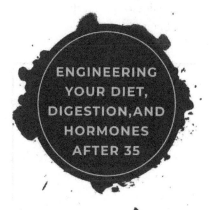

ENGINEERING YOUR DIET, DIGESTION, AND HORMONES AFTER 35

Dr. Jennifer Stagg

SAVIO
REPVBLIC

A SAVIO REPUBLIC BOOK
An Imprint of Post Hill Press
ISBN: 978-1-64293-282-9
ISBN (eBook): 978-1-64293-283-6

The Bitter Prescription:
Engineering Your Diet, Digestion, and Hormones After 35
© 2020 by Dr. Jennifer Stagg
All Rights Reserved

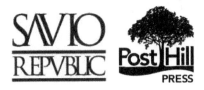

posthillpress.com
New York • Nashville
Published in the United States of America

*To my husband, Mark,
and my children, Ethan, Lilah, and Kate—
you inspire me to offer the best of myself to help make our world a
more loving and happy place. And to my beloved patients, who have
taught me more than they ever know, I am eternally grateful.*

Contents

Introduction ix

● **Section 1. Knowledge for the Bitter Prescription**

Chapter 1: Aging 3
Chapter 2: Digestive Health.. 17
Chapter 3: Eating 39
Chapter 4: Bitters... 47
Chapter 5: Hormonal Balance.. 61

● **Section 2. The Bitter Prescription Dietary Plan**

Chapter 6: Fat Loss... 83
Chapter 7: The Bitter Prescription Dietary Essentials 91
Chapter 8: The Bitter Prescription Foods........................... 103
Chapter 9: Menu Planning 133
Chapter 10: Recipes 137
Chapter 11: Nutritional Supplements................................. 157

● **Section 3. Executing the Bitter Prescription**

Chapter 12: Lifestyle Change and Compliance.................... 167
Chapter 13: Bitter Feelings.. 171
Chapter 14: Positive Mindset.. 187

My personal message to you 194

Introduction

For as long as I can remember, I have had a thirst for knowledge. I always wanted to know *why?* I collected information. In the beginning, informally, just storing it in the back of my mind, and then formally, legitimately amassing a real collection as my education evolved. The focus of my collection has always been factors involved in what makes people function better, mentally, emotionally, and physically, as well as living longer, healthier lives. I really wanted to know how I could operate at 100 percent and have the best chance of living a long life while feeling the best that I could.

As a teenager, I would watch health-related television programs and PBS specials and read magazine articles. I started to collect books, and as my education expanded, I attended lectures, read journal articles, and continued to add to my collection. I was always intrigued by centenarians, people who lived over one hundred years, and was completely fascinated when Dan Buettner's book, *The Blue Zones*, came out, detailing hot spots around the globe where clusters of people enjoyed long and healthy lives.

Once I became a physician, I was not only interested in better understanding the factors that accounted for longevity for my own personal interest, but now I was charged with helping to manage the health and well-being of other people. It became critical that I identify the most important lifestyle elements that contribute to healthspan, which is a term that refers to how long people live in a very good functioning state of health.

As I passed the forty-year mark, my interest in the science of aging really ramped up. During my first year in private practice, I realized that the majority of my patients were in the forty-to-sixty-year-old age range, so I had plenty of experience dealing with the clinical effects of aging in my practice. I also commonly heard patients remark to me, "Ever since I turned 'a certain age' [typically between thirty-five to forty], it's been downhill from there." Now in my early forties, I was also getting a close-up and personal experience with aging myself. With my unique clinical training, I worked diligently to identify the root causes of aging through reviews of evidence-based research, and in my practice, I had the ability to explore this further. Notably, in the setting of my clinic, I noticed two common factors that appeared to propel the aging process in my patients: specific dietary habits and emotional stress.

Clearly apparent, and indisputable, is the foundational effect of nutrition on longevity. However, in the data there is so much controversy about the finer details of diet and human health. The more one digs, the more conflicting data arises. With my undergraduate degree in nutritional biochemistry and having completed further graduate work in biochemistry, I felt I had been very well trained to weed though the wealth of information in the database.

Reading research studies is one thing. Working with actual people is a very different matter. We humans are extremely complex organisms. The ability to transfer what is learned in the scientific arena to individuals is not as simple as just handing out a food list and saying, "Here's your new diet. Just eat this way from now on." There is an art to working with people. The complexities of mindset and emotional well-being also need to be recognized and addressed.

Over the years, as I gained clinical experience in my practice, it became very clear to me that there were key factors in the dietary and lifestyle habits and mindset that made the biggest difference to the health outcomes I saw in my patients.

I saw firsthand that it really does matter what you eat and how much you eat. I discovered that the health of the digestive system greatly affected a person's response to a healthful diet. I had many patients who ate a seemingly healthy diet but still had nutritional deficiencies and imbalances resulting from insufficient dietary absorption of nutritional components of food. Then, on the other end of the spectrum, despite some popular arguments to the contrary, I also had never found anyone to exercise themselves into better shape while neglecting to follow a healthy diet. As I work with patients in my clinical practice, I am continually reminded of the quote by Hippocrates, "All disease begins in the gut." The two most common places I start with patients are assessment of digestive function and discussion of emotional health. Research is showing that these two are tightly connected. In fact, the complex nervous network in the gut is often referred to as the second brain.

Then there is the issue of aging and its effect on digestive capacity. Many patients visit me for advice on how to lose weight. Oftentimes they have tried many diets, and they are getting lack-luster results. In the earlier years, I didn't realize the one common thread that ran through many of these cases. Finally, it became apparent to me, and is of such critical importance that I knew that, if I could help them with this, it could change the entire course of their health. I came to the realization that most of them had the same complaint: not just the frustration with difficulty losing weight, but the common piece of information they provided is, "Since I turned X years old, what worked for me no longer works." Some physiologic change associated with their age appeared to be the trigger. They would tell me that they hadn't changed their diet or activity level but just started gaining weight. They said that there weren't any books or good information out there that advised people how to eat as they got older. For others who had participated in the cycle of dieting and lost the same twenty to thirty pounds over and over, they complained that dieting no longer worked. Of course, I added this information to my "collection" that I started way back in my teens, considering this information to be the most important element I had discovered yet.

Now, you may be identifying with this weight issue and wondering if there is hope, and let me tell you, "Yes, there is hope!" This book is a summation of my "collection" and what I have deduced, from many years in clinical practice, to be the most important factors that keep people in top-notch shape. I actually toyed with calling this book, "An eating guide for people over thirty-five" because I have discovered that our nutritional needs change quite a bit as we age, and you will learn all about it in this book.

The title I settled on is a reflection of the core elements of my prescription for better health as you age. First, the foods you must eat to improve your digestion and overall wellness. These foods fall into the nutritional category of dietary bitters and are packed with bioactive compounds that improve cellular health and metabolism. Second, the "bitter truth" about eating as you get older. This piece of advice does not win me any popularity contests, but it must be followed to attain results. If you have excess body fat stores, you need to eat less. It's simple, but I have found it very hard for people to hear—and even harder to execute. And third, the state of your emotional health matters and affects the aging process at least equally to dietary habits, if not more. Bitter feelings like resentment, irritability, anger, and pessimism can directly sabotage your health and keep you from leading a healthy lifestyle.

This is not the prescription a lot of people are ready to take, but it is my *Bitter Prescription*:

1. You need to eat less as you get older

2. Consume a variety of bitter foods in your diet regularly

3. Get rid of your bitter feelings

A lot of people find it much easier to just take a pill instead of dealing with themselves, working on their emotional health, and eating mindfully and healthfully while managing their digestive health.

I am sharing all of this with you because there is so much information out there. I constantly hear from my patients and friends that they don't know what to believe. As a result, they just continue to do the same and see the same results. What bothers them deeply is they know they should feel better than they do. They don't know where to start and often have a perception that the road to get there will be too difficult.

My wish for you is that you reach the point where you feel that you are the best possible version of yourself. And most importantly, I want this feeling to last throughout your entire life. I want to help you achieve your best chance of living a long and healthy life. That is the part that is the biggest issue in health and wellness today. Maintaining those healthy habits is the part that fails in most cases.

This book doesn't just detail another trendy diet. This is a lifestyle plan. I have arranged it into three sections so that you understand:

1. The knowledge behind what you should be doing to live a long healthy life, the *why*

2. The bitter prescription dietary plan, the *what* you should do

3. Execution, the *how* to do it, which addresses emotional well-being and mindset, how to banish bitter feelings, and how to attain better results to last

By following this three-step approach you have a better chance at success, far beyond what you have experienced in the past. It is my deepest desire that you reach the place where you feel your best, you are thriving, and you can share your unique gifts with our world so that we are all better for it.

With gratitude and love,
Jen

SECTION 1

Knowledge for the Bitter Prescription

CHAPTER 1

Aging

$\mathcal{W}$e are all aging from the moment we are born. While we are infants and children, we are developing and growing more bone and muscle, our organs are getting larger and we are making new neural connections. This type of aging is all viewed as a wonderful rite of passage. The time period that is viewed to have a negative connotation is that of our mid-to-late adult years. Most people begin to notice the effects of aging in their thirties. This is the age when patients start remarking to me that they are concerned about changes in their physical bodies and metabolic function, asking if the symptoms they are experiencing are just the product of getting older.

With all the developments in modern medicine, as of now, there is no way to stop the aging process. If someone figures out how to do that, it will be the most remarkable discovery of all time. As of now, we are all in the same boat. However, we do know that the rate at which we age can be accelerated, and it can be slowed down. Aging is affected by both genetics and lifestyle.

Genetic theories on aging are complex and require much more research. There is a rare genetic disorder, Hutchinson-Gilford progeria syndrome (HGPS), which results in rapid aging in children and, sadly, those affected usually don't live past thirteen years of age. Conditions like this give researchers an opportunity to study genetics, metabolism, and aging.

The lifestyle factors that impact aging have become much better understood. Stress and emotional health play a role in the process of aging, as do environmental chemicals, diet, and exercise. The overall approach to health care that I practice in my clinic emphasizes the importance of addressing all of these issues. If someone is coming in and their main concern is difficulty losing weight, we are going to be discussing not just diet and exercise but also their emotional health and how they are reacting to stressors in their lives.

⬤ PHYSICAL SIGNS AND SYMPTOMS OF AGING

If you've not yet experienced any effects of aging, you certainly know what to expect. Even little kids know what aging looks like and are not shy to point it out. My kids had no problem telling me about the lines around my eyes and how that is the defining feature that makes me look much older than them. The bitter truth here is that these signs and symptoms all suck! You know the themes of those memes: "I wish I looked and felt much older…said no one ever over the age of thirty-five!" Nobody wishes for thinning hair and memory problems.

Here are some of the major features associated with aging. I divided these into two categories: first, the appearance of aging and second, the feelings commonly associated with aging.

Appearance and signs associated with aging:

* slowed wound and injury healing
* ridges in nails
* wrinkles and crow's feet
* age spots
* loose and thinning skin
* sagging buttocks and breasts
* thickening of skin on heels
* spider veins and varicosities
* gray hair

* thinning hair
* lack of luster in hair
* cellulite
* loss of height
* more fat in midsection
* loss of muscle mass

How you feel/the symptoms associated with aging:

* joint pain
* reduced flexibility
* memory issues
* poor mental stamina
* lack of focus
* need for reading glasses (presbyopia)
* poor exercise tolerance
* muscle weakness and soreness
* tired
* insomnia and sleeping problems
* waking feeling unrested
* low libido

WHAT MAKES US AGE

A combination of factors contributes to the aging process, including genetics and how those genes are influenced by diet, lifestyle, and the environment, which is collectively referred to as epigenetics, the effect of external factors on DNA. *Epi* is a Greek prefix that means *above* or *on.* The sequence of DNA doesn't change. Instead, genes can get turned on or off. These changes can have a profound impact on our health and can get passed on to our children, and even through multiple generations. This was covered extensively in my last book, *Unzip Your Genes*. The good news is that epigenetic effects are reversible, and that's what this book is about. You have the power to change how your DNA gets expressed through how you live—your daily lifestyle choices.

These epigenetic signatures, including DNA methylation and microRNAs, can be affected by a wide spectrum of environmental factors, including smoking, exercise, psychological stress, sleep, drugs, and nutrition. Consequently, aging and resultant conditions may have strong switch-like epigenetic origins in gene regulation. We know that even simple changes like taking B vitamins and following a Mediterranean-style diet can reverse altered epigenetic patterns in genes related to energy metabolism and inflammation.

Premature aging
Which factors speed up the aging process and accelerate the incidence of age-related diseases? There are some known genetic factors at play, but, for most of us, lifestyle is the key regulator of aging. Stress is arguably the most important accelerator of aging. Have you seen side-by-side photos of US presidents before and after they served their four-year term? The physical changes are dramatic and clearly demonstrate the impact of stress. Lack of sleep is another driver of premature aging. We also know that people who smoke experience rapid aging, and significant exposure to other environmental chemicals also speeds up the aging process. One of the biggest problems facing Americans is the obesity epidemic, and this also can negatively impact core processes involved in accelerated aging. Excess fatty tissue changes DNA expression, and these epigenetic modifications impact genes related to inflammation, cholesterol and fat metabolism, and type 2 diabetes. In this

chapter, I will cover how important it is to reduce excess belly fat, and in the second part of this book, I will discuss just how to do this. Difficulty losing belly fat as they get older has been a common complaint from many of my patients.

Can we slow it down or turn back the clock?

The short answer is yes, without a doubt. The evidence to date completely supports the effect of a healthy lifestyle in aging. These factors have been extensively studied by Dr. Frank Hu's research group at Harvard T.H. Chan School of Public Health, and the consensus on slowing down the aging process and reducing chronic disease risk—coronary heart disease (80 percent lower), type 2 diabetes (90 percent lower), cancer (40–60 percent lower), and stroke (40–50 percent lower)—includes these five low-risk lifestyle factors:

1. Physical activity—more than 3.5 hrs. per week

2. Consuming a healthy diet—(top 40 percent alternative healthy eating index)

3. Moderate alcohol consumption—females 5–15 g/day and males 5–20 g/day

4. Maintaining a healthy weight—defined by Body Mass Index (BMI) of 18.5–24.9 kg/m^2

5. Non-smoker

The sad part is that only 3–4 percent of subjects in the study group actually followed all five factors of the low-risk healthy lifestyle. The silver lining here is that there is so much opportunity to work with most of the population to improve overall health and longevity. A recent report estimated life expectancy when starting from age fifty, and for women who followed none of the factors on the list, they could expect to live until seventy-nine years of age, while women who had all five of these factors could expect to live fourteen years longer, until the age of ninety-three. For men, this same trend was increased from seventy-five to eighty-seven years of age.

➾ COMPRESSION OF MORBIDITY

Who wants to live to one hundred and spend the last twenty to thirty years dealing with health problems that interfere with your ability to enjoy life? The concept of compression of morbidity comes from the research community and is used to study health trends. The chronic ailments and illnesses that pop up as we get older (morbidity just means the presence of illness) are associated with the aging process. Inevitably, we will all die. However, if we die of "old age," ideally our health status only declines rapidly, close to the end of life. That is what is meant by compression of morbidity.

➾ WHAT IS INFLAMMAGING?

I often describe the very act of getting older as a mild inflammatory state. Aging is characterized by an imbalance between inflammatory and anti-inflammatory responses to all our external stressors. The concern here is not just the appearance of more lines on your face. Chronic inflammation is a risk factor for morbidity and mortality in the elderly. It's also a major determinant of global aging and longevity in general. *Inflammaging*, as it is called, and its accompanying loss of immune function helps explain the increased incidence in age-related diseases, since most chronic diseases share an inflammatory origin.

Basics on inflammation and oxidation

Chronic inflammation and oxidative stress are thought to accelerate aging, consequently influencing longevity and health. The key regulatory molecule for inflammation is NF-κB. When we study naturally occurring chemicals in our food called bioactives, many of which are also bitter compounds, we see how they can reduce NF-κB. A potent NF-κB inhibitor is curcumin, a bitter bioactive found in the culinary spice turmeric. Similarly, these bioactive compounds can also act as direct antioxidants, scavenging reactive oxygen species (ROS) that can damage our DNA. These bitter bioactives can also result in changes that impact another molecule called NRF2, which is the key regulator of oxidation. The processes of inflammation and oxidative stress are tightly linked, with each stimulating the other, thereby creating a vicious cycle. Again, the good news here is that our lifestyle choices, including chemical exposures and psychological and physical stress, impact both inflammation and oxidative stress and, in turn, aging. We can actively change the course of our health trajectory and lifespan.

Sources of inflammation

Inducers of the inflammatory cascade are generated from outside (exogenous) and inside (endogenous) the body. For example, eating a diet filled with inflammatory foods can trigger inflammation. People who are experiencing pain often take anti-inflammatory medications or, in my practice, use anti-inflammatory supplements like curcumin. They may also switch to an anti-inflammatory diet if they are eating foods that could trigger inflammation, and that may settle it down, reducing the need for medication. However, if they have excess belly fat, also called visceral adipose tissue (VAT), which acts like an organ that produces a constant flow of inflammatory signals, no matter how clean their diet is and how many anti-inflammatories they take, they will not get rid of the chronic inflammation. This is why reducing excess belly fat is so important.

Resolution of inflammation

When I talk to my patients about inflammation, I often talk about putting out the fire. The general approach to inflammation has been focused on treatment with anti-inflammatory agents, whether synthetic or naturally derived. It turns out that is not the entire story. We now know there is another phase of the inflammatory process called the resolution phase. This stage involves a separate, active pathway other than the initiation pathway. The way I approach inflammation in my practice has changed dramatically. While I still address inflammatory triggers that result in changes in DNA methylation patterns (including helping patients get rid of excess belly fat), I also use targeted supplementation in the form of specialized pro-resolving mediators, better known as SPMs. SPMs are made in our body from dietary omega-3 fatty acids, and they stimulate the resolution phase of inflammation, which ultimately turns off chronic inflammation. As we get older, we don't make SPMs in our bodies very effectively. If we have excess belly fat, we do even worse. Therefore, supplementing with SPMs can be a good way to quell the fire of inflammation that could accelerate aging.

ARE THERE BIOMARKERS FOR AGING?

Although not used in clinical practice yet, there are some very accurate calculations to predict age that are based on testing for epigenetic changes on DNA. These can be thought of as an epigenetic clock and can even predict risk of early death. These calculations result in a value called the "methylation age" or "mAge," and the two used in research are the Hannum age predictor and the Horvath age predictor. mAge can be higher as a result of dietary and lifestyle factors such as low consumption of fish, fruits, and vegetables, minimal exercise, and even low income or education levels.

Bone and muscle mass loss are associated with healthspan
Musculoskeletal deterioration results from the slowing down of bone turnover and muscle building. As we get older, we can experience a progressive loss of muscle mass which, when deficient, is referred to as sarcopenia. It takes a higher amount of protein intake to synthesize the same amount of muscle as a younger adult, which is known as anabolic resistance. This process is influenced by depressed immune function and chronic inflammation, which is characteristic of aging. We also know that, as adults age, there is a reduced ability to digest and absorb protein, and often a lower intake of protein due to a reduction in appetite. Poor dental health, problems with swallowing, side effects of medicines, and social isolation become more impactful issues as we advance in age.

Not only does sarcopenia result in loss of mobility and physical performance, but it's also associated with many of the chronic health problems that afflict us as we get older, including:

* increased inflammation
* hormone imbalance
* psychological changes, especially depression
* mental/cognitive conditions
* increased risk of infection and fever
* increased incidence of falls
* more surgeries

Chronic inflammatory response syndrome (CIRS)
A more extreme example of the effect of chronic inflammation is in the case of people who have a condition called CIRS. As the result of identified genetic factors, inflammation can stay "turned on" in up to 20 percent of the population. I commonly see this condition play out in patients who visit me who were infected with tick-borne illnesses like Lyme disease. In these

patients, exposure to an infection can ignite the inflammatory cascade, and innate immunity doesn't get turned off. About 80 percent of people who have had Lyme disease tend to have no ill effects after the infection has cleared, but 20 percent still do, and those are thought be the ones with CIRS. There are more than thirty identifiable triggers (biotoxins), including mold exposure. Fortunately, there is hope for people affected by CIRS, and working with a health care provider who understands this condition can offer a path to recovery.

➡ DIET AND AGING

Dietary requirements change as you age. Our digestive systems become less effective at digesting and assimilating nutrients into your tissues. This is why nutrient deficiencies are more common as people get older, and it also contributes to body composition changes as people lose muscle and bone mass with age. On average, these changes can start as early as thirty-five years of age. In my clinical practice, this is the age group in which I tend to observe more digestive problems, as well. Digestive health will be covered in more detail in the next chapter.

How to get results with dietary changes?

Almost everyone who comes to my clinic asks the same question in relation to almost every health complaint they have: "Is there something I could do with my diet that would help me?" When it comes to the aging process and metabolism, the answer is clearly yes. You may be surprised, but the first thing I recommend is what I have found to be the most important piece of knowledge you need to know to maintain good health as you age. (You may have guessed it because I have already mentioned it many times in this chapter.) If you are retaining excess stores of body fat, then getting rid of that excess fat is a top priority. And as we get older, one of the most important factors that plays a role here is the amount of fuel, or calories, you consume daily. The bitter truth that most people don't like to hear is that you are going to need to eat less calories than you currently consume in order to reduce your body fat. There are so many diet and nutrition experts out there saying that calories no longer matter and that you don't have to think about the portion sizes of the food you eat. That is simply not true. It sounds great to have no limit on the amount of food you can eat. That's why many people find those food plans to be so attractive, but they end up failing when it comes to results if you are overeating and exceeding the number of calories required for your body's needs. You're probably wondering more about exactly how much less, and I will address this. And, of course, it goes without saying, you also need to eat nutritious foods, rich in bitter bioactive compounds (I will also get to this as you read on). You can't expect to feel better, improve your metabolism, and slow down the aging process on a diet of processed food, devoid of nutrients, typical of the Standard American Diet.

The effect of excess body fat
Just one word can sum this one up: inflammation. If you have too much fat stored in your body, this is potentially the number one driver of chronic inflammation. And as you know, inflammation promotes premature aging. Visceral belly fat provides cushioning for your organs but also acts like its own organ of inflammation, secreting chemical messages that keep the inflammatory process smoldering. To make matters worse, as we age, we also have difficulty resolving inflammation, so there is not an effective "off switch."

Why you need to reduce your body fat
Simply put, as you reduce the amount of excess fat stored in your body, inflammation levels may follow suit. I have seen this time and again with patients in my clinic. We use body composition

testing that shows how much fat is stored in the body, and it even details where it resides: trunk, arms, and legs. This allows us to reliably assess how much of the changes in body weight on a standard scale are the result of fat loss versus muscle and water loss. Laboratory testing can track biomarkers for inflammation, like C-reactive protein, and I often observe those trending downward when a person is shedding excess stored belly fat. If inflammatory markers are not declining, there may be other factors involved, and we may need to do additional diagnostic testing to explore what else may be going on in that case.

Caloric intake as you age

When you are young and still in a state of growth, referred to as an anabolic, or building, state, your body requires more calories than when you are fully grown and have transitioned to a catabolic state where, unfortunately, your body is slowly breaking down. This explains why women often come to me saying that they have eaten the same way for many years and haven't changed their exercise levels, but they just slowly continue to gain weight. The bitter truth is that, because they are getting older, they now have to change their diet to adapt to the changes in metabolism that accompany age. They have to eat less calories and be selective about where those calories are coming from.

Not too long ago, I had a male patient, who is in his seventies and is in excellent health (and has one of the best advanced cholesterol profiles I have ever seen at any age) remark to me that he is surprised how little food he eats now compared to how he ate when he was younger, yet he is still satisfied and has plenty of energy to lead an active lifestyle. When my mother asked me what this book was about and I started explaining the three main tenets of my "Bitter Prescription," when I told her that people need to eat less as they age, she said that was absolutely true and remarked that she feels much better eating less than she did when she was younger and believes she is able to maintain a healthy weight by eating less.

The truth is that, as we reach "a certain age," we really do need to reduce the number of calories coming in. This doesn't necessarily mean the *amount* of food needs to be reduced, because we can change the *composition* of our diets. Simply put, we can eat more nutrient-rich foods like vegetables, beans, and fruit, which contain less calories and reduce our intake of calorie-rich foods like processed carbs, fatty meats, oils, and so on. Furthermore, we can also structure our daily meal times and order of eating and include more foods that are rich in bitter bioactives to improve our digestion and metabolism.

The evidence on eating 300 calories less per day
A recent study conducted at Duke University set out to look at the health outcomes of patients with metabolic syndrome when they reduced their dietary intake by 300 calories per day. Metabolic syndrome is an increasingly common condition defined by meeting at least three of five criteria: high blood pressure, high blood sugar, high triglycerides, low HDL cholesterol, and excess belly fat. They divided the subjects into two groups and tracked them for two years. The group on the lower-calorie diet, on average, lost about sixteen pounds, mostly from belly fat, and improved all their other biomarkers studied. To date, caloric restriction has been shown to increase lifespan in all types of animals studied, as well as improve overall healthspan, which is also known as compression of morbidity (discussed earlier in this chapter).

CHAPTER 2

Digestive Health

*H*ow many people do you know who complain of digestive problems, whether occasionally or most of the time? Everything from stomachaches, nausea, heartburn, indigestion, bloating, constipation, and diarrhea to full-blown diagnosed medical conditions like ulcerative colitis and Crohn's disease. Digestive complaints are some of the most common symptoms that people experience, and in my clinical practice, I see evidence of that every day. In fact, about 75 percent of people complain of some sort of digestive issue.

During my medical training, I was first introduced to the famous concept heralded by Hippocrates: all disease begins in the gut. Basically, this theory implicates dysfunction in the digestive tract as playing a key role in the origin and development of chronic health problems. In recent years, publications in scientific journals have begun to support this theory, especially with the tremendous amount of ongoing research on the microbiome (the bacteria in the gut) and the role of inflammation in the gut. These disturbances can cause digestive symptoms but have also been linked to a broad range of problems, everything from weight gain to diabetes, autoimmune diseases, and conditions in the nervous system.

➥ COMMON GASTROINTESTINAL (GI) COMPLAINTS

Patients can exhibit a broad range of GI symptoms that can correlate with a variety of clinical conditions, making diagnosis challenging for the clinician. These are the most common symptoms people report:

* Constipation ✓
* Diarrhea ✓
* Loose stools ✓
* Bowel urgency ✓
* Eructation
* Excessive flatulence ✓
* Foul-smelling gas
* Halitosis (Bad breath)
* Abdominal pain or spasm
* Abdominal distension/bloating ✓
* Hemorrhoids ✓
* Change in stool size, color, consistency
* Blood or mucus in stool
* Heartburn ✓
* Indigestion
* Nausea, vomiting

To further complicate the clinical picture, some patients with diagnosed diseases such as celiac disease may be successfully managing their disease but could be having symptoms from another GI condition, and their concerns may be dismissed as just part of the known diagnosis. Multiple GI conditions can be present at the same time, so it is really important to work with a skilled diagnostician. Then there are "silent" GI conditions like intestinal permeability, and some patients can have symptoms in other body systems that are the result of GI issues such as in the case of silent reflux and sinusitis, or in hypochlorhydria (low stomach acid) and rosacea.

Why are digestive problems so common?

The most obvious explanation is our diet. Over the last seventy-five years, our diet has changed dramatically, but our bodies can't evolve that quickly to keep up with this type of environmental change. Not only have we transitioned to eating more processed and genetically modified food, our food is also shipped from all over the world, which impacts the food quality. Our soils have become depleted of many important nutrients so that even regionally grown produce often isn't as nutritious as it was fifty years ago. Furthermore, we are stressed to the max, often eating on the run, which can impact our ability to digest food and the health of our microbiome. Then, to add fuel to the fire, our environment is abundant with toxic chemicals that can impact gut health.

➡ AGING AND DIGESTIVE HEALTH

Digestive complaints become more common as we age. As I explained in the last chapter, when we are older, our overall metabolism is in a state of decline. Diagnosis of diseases of the gastrointestinal tract are much more prevalent in people over forty. Risks of nutritional deficiencies go up with age. People tend to notice more issues with foods that seem to bother them in some way, in some causing heartburn or indigestion, while others feel certain meals tend to just sit heavy in their stomach. Bloating is a common complaint I hear in my clinical practice, especially in women over thirty-five. An extremely common complaint with aging is constipation, as the bowel becomes more sluggish. Most seniors take a fiber supplement for regularity.

Higher risk of nutrient deficiencies with age

As we age, especially over fifty, our risk of having vitamin and mineral deficiencies goes up. In my clinical practice, I definitely observe increased rates of nutrient deficiency as people get older, but I routinely see it in people in their late thirties and early forties, too. While deficiency states can often result from lack of those nutrients in the diet, in the case of the aging adult, reduced digestive capacity can play a larger role. It is well established that, as we get older, the body becomes less efficient at absorbing nutrients from food, which makes it even more important to eat food that is rich in healthy nutrients.

A classic example of this is vitamin B12 deficiency in older individuals, which is most commonly the result of low stomach acid production, referred to as hypochlorhydria (more in this section), and *Helicobacter pylori* infection in the stomach. The Institute of Medicine recommends that people over fifty should take synthetic B12 supplements because, unlike food, this form of B12 is unbound and better able to be absorbed. The symptoms of B12 deficiency can include mood changes and memory problems, fatigue, anemia, muscle weakness, nerve issues, shakiness, and even incontinence. Vitamin B12 is very important for the nervous system, making new red blood cells, and DNA production. This is just one clear example of how a vitamin deficiency can impact many body systems. Vitamin B12 deficiency can be screened for with a simple blood test.

Most common nutritional deficiencies for people over fifty

Aside from vitamin B12 deficiency, there are quite a few other vitamin and mineral deficiencies to watch out for as we get older. These include:

* Calcium

* Folate

* Magnesium

* Potassium

* Vitamin B6

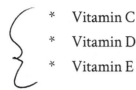

* Vitamin C
* Vitamin D
* Vitamin E

Compromised digestion and nutrient deficiency

Let's take a more extreme case, gastric bypass surgery, in which absorption in the gut is significantly affected. The most common deficiencies in people who have had this type of weight loss surgery are vitamin B12, folate, zinc, iron, copper, calcium, and vitamin D. As a result, they are at higher risk of developing other medical problems like osteoporosis, anemia, and neuropathy in their hands and feet.

Another example of the impact of compromised digestive capacity is in the long-term use of a class of stomach acid-suppressing medications called proton pump inhibitors (PPIs). Research has shown that long-term PPI use increases the risk of vitamin B12, vitamin C, calcium, iron, and magnesium deficiencies. And to lend further support to the theory that diseases can start in the gut, PPIs are also linked to increased risk of fractures, pneumonia, chronic kidney disease, dementia, cardiovascular diseases, and a higher risk of premature death.

➡ LET'S TALK DIGESTION—THE BASICS

You must be digesting well for the nutritional components of food to get absorbed into your blood stream. Some components of food, like fiber, are meant to stay in the gut, and bitter bioactive compounds like curcuminoids and quercetin exert some of their effects in the intestinal environment, too. Adequate digestion is necessary for these small phytochemicals to be released from food. If food is not getting digested completely, then it's pretty likely gut bacteria is out of balance, too.

The entire digestive tract, from the mouth to the anus, is actually considered an external environment. The gut barrier separates and protects the internal environment. After food gets digested, in order for the smaller elements to be absorbed and enter the bloodstream, they must pass through channels or transporters in the intestinal cells to be delivered to different parts of the body.

Absorption is of critical importance to your health, because the nutrients and bioactives in food will eventually affect your DNA. This is the fundamental principle of nutrigenomics. We also know that bioactives in food are good for your gut bacteria. As I mentioned, 100 percent of food is not meant to be absorbed, and some of the bioactives can sit around in the intestines. This explains why components in turmeric have low rates of absorption, even in someone with very healthy digestive function.

Prior to food entering the intestines, there is a lot more digestive work that needs to occur to ultimately allow these smaller elements to be used in cellular metabolism. The digestive process can actually begin before food even enters your mouth. You may have heard about Pavlov's dog experiments, where he first discovered that dogs produced saliva in response to just hearing or smelling food. He later demonstrated that the dogs would produce saliva from a neutral sound that was associated with the feeding. You may have observed this in your home if you have a pet, when you open the cabinet door where the cat food is stored, and your kitty comes running. And we humans are no different. We can start salivating at the thought of food or actions associated with food. In the following section, I will detail the digestive process from the thought and smell of food, chewing, then through the stomach and intestines.

Phases of digestion
There are three main phases of digestion, the cephalic, gastric, and intestinal phases. The cephalic phase occurs before food even enters the mouth and can start with just the thought or

sound of food, and most certainly with the smell or sight of food. This is thought to be the pre-digestive component which prepares the body for incoming food. The brain signals the stomach, via the vagus nerve, to secrete gastric juices. Once you put food in your mouth, then digestion really gets going as you begin to mechanically break down your food by chewing it and coating it with saliva, which contains amylase, the first enzyme that makes contact with food. This enzyme starts the process of breaking down starch. Saliva is alkaline, and this environment is important for amylase to work efficiently.

Once food is swallowed, the gastric phase begins when food enters the stomach. Gastric juices containing stomach acid, specifically hydrochloric acid (HCl), and pepsin (an enzyme that digests protein) help digest food further, while the stomach (which is basically a big muscular chamber) churns and mechanically breaks down food until it becomes a substance referred to as chyme. Gastrin is a hormone in the stomach that triggers the release of acid and pepsin.

As chyme passes into the first part of the small intestine, called the duodenum, the intestinal phase of digestion begins. The arrival of chyme here signals the release of other digestive hormones, secretin and cholecystokinin (CCK), that stimulate the pancreas and gall bladder. The pancreas releases sodium bicarbonate, changing the acidity level in the duodenum, and digestive enzymes: pancreatic proteases (such as trypsin and chymotrypsin) which help digest proteins, pancreatic amylase which works on carbohydrates and pancreatic lipase that aids fat breakdown. The gallbladder releases bile which aids the digestion and absorption of dietary fats and fat-soluble vitamins. Two other digestive hormones are also released here: gastric inhibitory peptide (GIP), which can stimulate insulin production from the pancreas, and motilin, which effects motility of the intestinal tract. There are additional enzymes that sit on the brush border of the intestinal tract in those finger-like projections called villi: maltase-glucoamylase, sucrase-isomal-tase, lactase (for smaller carbohydrates), peptidases (smaller proteins), and lipases (fats). These are the enzymes that are affected when someone has celiac disease prior to treatment with a gluten-free diet.

You are probably starting to realize how complex the digestive process is; not something you really think of every time you eat an apple. That brings us to the appetite-regulatory hormones, which are:

* ghrelin, which is released from the stomach and reaches the pituitary gland and stimulates appetite

* PYY from the small intestine that counteracts ghrelin

* leptin from fat cells that targets the hypothalamus in the brain to reduce appetite

* adiponectin, also from fat cells, which can increase appetite

These hormones are the target of some obesity researchers, because increased leptin concentrations and decreased adiponectin and ghrelin may lead to a reduced appetite. There is much complexity regarding the roles of these hormones. I will discuss leptin and adiponectin more in the upcoming hormone chapter. They play an important role in fat and glucose metabolism.

As the bolus of food travels through the small intestine and is broken down into smaller components, absorption of nutrients becomes the focus. By the time it reaches the end of the small intestine, there is not much left to absorb, other than water and electrolytes. In the large intestine, water is reabsorbed as the stool is formed, which is composed of the remaining waste products, fiber, bacteria, and old, dead cells from the lining of the digestive tract.

➡ HOW IS YOUR DIGESTION?

When I am assessing digestive health for a patient, I consider five key areas, which I will cover in more detail next. These are:

1. Motility

2. Acid production

3. Enzymes and bile salts

4. Microbiome

5. Inflammation

Motility

By motility, I am referring to the rate at which food is moving through the intestinal tract. Most common, as we age, is slow motility. I can't even begin to guess how many times I have used the diagnosis code for "constipation due to slow transit time." The intestines can get sluggish with age, but sometimes slow motility is due to other imbalances such as inactivity, not drinking enough water, low-fiber diet, microbiome imbalance, stress, and hormonal issues such as hypothyroidism. I often assess how much dietary fiber and water a patient is consuming. Daily fiber intake should be in the range of 25–35 grams. Insoluble fiber tends to add bulk to stool. I am also selective about fiber sources. For example, along with being a good source of dietary fiber, prunes contain sorbitol, which draws water into the intestines, and phenolic compounds that support beneficial bacteria. Bitters come into play here as well. Bitter compounds interact with bitter taste receptors in the intestinal tract and can help regulate motility.

Sometimes intestinal motility can be increased, pushing everything through too quickly, often resulting in loose stools and diarrhea. This is commonly the result of dysregulated nerve function in the gut, impaired digestion, microbiome imbalance, food intolerances, and allergies or hormone problems. People with disordered motility can experience intestinal cramps or spasms and abdominal pain.

Acid production

Producing optimal levels of stomach acid, not too much and not too little, is critical for good digestive health. It is quite obvious for most people when they are producing too much acid, because they will feel symptoms of heartburn. Not as common, is a condition called silent reflux, which doesn't produce classic warmth or burning in the chest but can manifest as excess mucus in the upper throat area. Even less common is when people have symptoms of heartburn that actually may arise from a lower esophageal sphincter that is not closing down properly, which could be due to tissue changes or from low stomach acid that doesn't signal the sphincter to shut tightly. This situation is quite uncommon. You shouldn't make any assumptions on your own and start supplementing with acid pills, called betaine HCl, because it could cause damage to your stomach.

The bigger issue I want to address here is low stomach acid, referred to as hypochlorhydria. In most cases, the symptoms of this condition are not obvious, and unlike heartburn, most people have never even heard of this. However, as people age, they are more likely to be affected by hypochlorhydria. In fact, about 15 percent of people over the age of sixty-five have low stomach acid. Because the stomach plays such a key role in the digestion, if there is not enough acid being produced by the stomach cells, bigger problems can result downstream. Other causes of low stomach acid include chronic stress, low dietary intake of bitters, low intake of zinc and B vitamins, medications like proton pump inhibitors (PPIs), excessive alcohol use, stomach surgery like gastric bypass and *Helicobacter pylori* infection of the stomach.

Conditions associated with low stomach acid

* autoimmune diseases
* atopic disease—asthma, allergies, eczema
* chronic infections
* iron deficiency anemia
* skin problems like acne, psoriasis, rosacea
* osteoporosis
* thyroid disease

Common symptoms of low stomach acid

* thinning hair
* weak, brittle fingernails
* desire to eat when not hungry
* weight problems
* signs of advanced aging in skin—wrinkles, sagging, dusky appearance
* fatigue
* gas, bloating, burping, upset stomach, nausea
* undigested food in stool, diarrhea
* microbiome imbalance, SIBO
* vitamin and mineral deficiencies
* neurological symptoms like numbness and tingling

Are there medical tests for low stomach acid?

A diagnostic test we have used in our practice is called the Heidelberg pH test. It involves swallowing a capsule that measures the resting acid level, or pH, in your stomach. Then, the patient is given a small amount of baking soda, which is alkaline, to measure the response of the acid-producing cells in the stomach. Although this test may be more accurate, this type of diagnostic device is not widely available and can take a long time to perform, so it is much easier to try the home screening methods.

Home screening techniques for adequate acid

There are a couple of easy ways to screen for low stomach acid at home. The one I commonly recommend to my patients is the baking soda test. The beet test also screens for low stomach acid but can pick up problems with your microbiome.

Baking soda test

First thing in the morning, on an empty stomach, stir 1/4 tsp. of baking soda into 4 oz. of water until it is completely dissolved, then drink all at once. Set a timer and wait to see how long it takes to burp. If it takes more than two minutes to burp, it may indicate you have low stomach acid. If you burp right away, within the first thirty seconds, you may be producing too much acid.

Beet test

Have you ever been alarmed that you had blood in your urine, only to remember that you have just recently eaten beets? The compounds in beets that are responsible for their characteristic deep purple pigment are broken down by stomach acid and your gut bacteria.

If either of these is not adequate, you can end up with beeturia, where your urine turns pink or deeper red after you have eaten beets. This test is not specific for low stomach acid, because it can also be the result of an imbalanced microbiome. Either way, there is a digestive issue here that should be further assessed to understand what exactly is going on.

What can increase stomach acid?

Bitter herbal blends, which often contain gentian, can be an effective way to kickstart sluggish stomach cells to produce more acid. These herbs are taken prior to the start of a meal to stimulate the bitter receptors that can then upregulate gastric acid production. If you have a history of peptic ulcer disease, bitter medical plant formulas should be avoided. In this case, I tend to work with dietary therapy and use other effective plant medicines to help heal and nourish the stomach and intestinal lining.

Should you start taking betaine HCl pills with meals?

There are quite a few reasons why HCl pills may not be advisable and could result in harm, so it is best you speak with a knowledgeable, integrative physician to make sure you are a good candidate for taking this supplement. For example, if you take NSAIDs, you should not use betaine HCl, as it could increase the risk of a gastrointestinal bleed. Also, if you have certain conditions of the GI tract, including ulcers and inflammation, you should also steer clear of supplemental acid.

Enzymes and bile salts

Diagnostic testing can reveal whether someone is having an issue with low pancreatic enzyme function. In that case, it's easy to supplement with oral pancreatic enzymes that are meant to be taken with each meal to aid digestion. If the problem is with enzymes secreted from the lining of the intestinal tract, then non-pancreatic origin digestive enzymes may provide support for improving digestive capacity. Increasing the intake of dietary bitters can also help.

I have also observed bile salts to be tremendously valuable in people who have had their gallbladder removed. While many who have had this type of surgery experience no problems with digestion, some suffer from chronic diarrhea or loose stools, especially after eating a fatty meal. They can also be prone to deficiencies in fat-soluble vitamins due to the malabsorption that may result. Taking bile salts with meals can address these issues.

What is the role of the microbiota in digestion?
Gut bacteria have many roles, including helping with the digestion and assimilation of food. These bacteria even produce secondary bile acids that assist with the absorption of dietary fats and fat-soluble vitamins like vitamin A and vitamin E. I have found that people who have had their gall bladder removed and have a healthy microbiota tend to have less issues with digesting fats.

The gut microbiota also plays a role in healthy cellular regeneration of the cells lining the intestinal tract to maintain a good gut barrier, as well as in immune function and mediating inflammatory processes. Without a strong barrier, bacterial byproducts and even bacteria can migrate into circulation, and in severe systemic situations, such as burns, major surgery, or trauma, can even cause sepsis.

Which factors influence the health of the microbiota?

1. Stress is a continued theme and cause of health problems that comes up in virtually every chronic health problem. It is one of the main underlying reasons for visits to the doctor's office.

2. Certain classes of medications are known to be a predisposing factor in the development of a condition known as SIBO (small intestinal bacterial overgrowth) which is characterized by an excess of inappropriate bacterial species in the small intestine. Bacteria that should reside in the large intestine can translocate, moving further up the intestinal tract to the small intestine, and set up camp. The most common symptoms in people with SIBO include diarrhea, abdominal pain, and bloating, although a wide variety of symptoms can be associated with it, including heartburn, chest pain, nausea, belching, flatulence, and constipation. A meta-analysis study showed that one third of people with irritable bowel syndrome (IBS) tested positive for SIBO. The most common test for SIBO is the lactulose breath test, which measures levels of hydrogen and methane gas produced by bacteria in the small intestine. The classes of medication that have been implicated in this condition include proton pump inhibitors, antibiotics, opiates, and anticholinergics.

Other risk factors that predispose to SIBO include:

*   hypochlorhydria

*   chronic pancreatitis

*   common variable immunodeficiency (CVID)

*   connective tissue disease (such as scleroderma)

*   diabetes mellitus

*   medications (opiates, anticholinergics)

*   post-operative adhesions

*   small bowel diverticula and strictures

      *   incompetent ileocecal valve

3.   Exercise plays a role in maintaining a healthy micro-biota. In fact, recent research has shown that there is a significant difference in the types and counts of bacteria in women who are sedentary versus those who lead an active lifestyle. They were even able to demonstrate improvements in the microbiota for women who broke out of the sedentary lifestyle.

4.   Infections can really upset the balance of bacteria in the microbiome. Having a gastrointestinal illness caused by a virus or from foodborne illness can wreak havoc, the effects lasting long after the infection is gone. I have seen many patients with microbiome imbalance that we can track back to an intestinal infection.

5.   Dietary factors are well known to impact the health of the microbiome. Diversity of the types of commensal bacteria found in the gut is the hallmark of a healthy microbiome. Consuming a wide variety of plants in the diet is the key feature that is associated with microbial diversity, especially eating a diet rich in plants that contain pre-biotic fiber and other bioactive compounds that regulate healthy commensal bacteria in the gut. Simply put, greater diversity of plants in the diet equates to improved microbial diversity.

Which problem comes first, digestive dysfunction or microbiome imbalance?

Even if you are eating a diet rich in plants, it may still lack vital nutrients and bioactives due to industrial agriculture and modernization of the food supply (including debittering, which I will cover in the chapter on bitters). This can impact the health of the microbiome. As I mentioned, gut bacteria also help with digestion of food in the intestinal tract. Poor digestion in the stomach when there is not enough stomach acid present can also impact the health of the microbiome. So which comes first? Chicken or egg? Primarily, the microbiome is affected by what food is coming in and how well it is processed before it hits the intestines. But as you will learn, the quality of food you consume not only affects the microbiome in the intestines, it can impact digestion in the stomach through lack of bitter bioactive compounds to bind the bitter taste receptors and impact digestive capacity.

Microbiome balance and food cravings
Did you know that it is well established that bacteria that reside in your gut have the ability to "speak" to your brain and influence your cravings for sugary foods that can promote their growth? I know when I first read these studies, I was somewhat shocked to learn that these bacteria can release toxins that can affect our mood, causing us to crave foods that are high in sugar or fat to fuel their growth. They also can make us feel happy through changing our taste buds, releasing neurotransmitters like serotonin and dopamine, which make us feel good, and even increasing the expression of cannabinoid and opiate receptors to reward us for eating the foods they want. Make no wonder, we can feel like food cravings have overtaken our system and have a sense of loss of control.

Inflammation in the digestive tract
Diagnostic testing can reveal inflammation in the gut. If that is a finding on the test panel, then my primary goal is to first identify and treat the root cause of inflammation in the gut

instead of only recommending anti-inflammatories. Similar to the concept of reducing excess body fat as a source of inflammation, we want to determine what could be causing the inflammation in the gut and address that first. For example, increased fiber intake has been shown to reduce inflammation and pain in osteoarthritis. There are theories that suggest obesity may actually start in the gut as intestinal inflammation and cause deposition of visceral fat, preceding the development of obesity, insulin resistance, diabetes, and chronic pain.

The most common sources of gut inflammation fall into four main categories:

1. Dietary sources: overall composition of the diet, food allergies, food sensitivities

2. Microbiome dysbiosis and resultant production of endotoxins

3. Environmental exposures, oxidative stress, prescription medicines

4. Emotional stress resulting in a gut bacterial shift with higher counts of bacteria producing inflammatory signals and lower counts of bacteria that are anti-inflammatory (a pattern described in inflammatory bowel disease)

How does stress effect the digestive system?

When you are under acute stress and your fight-or-flight response system has been turned on, intestinal contractions speed up and blood flow is shunted away from the digestive system to prepare you to run or engage in battle. This process impacts all aspects of digestive function. And, as I just mentioned, emotional stress increases inflammation in the gut through changes in the microbiota.

Digestive rest and why it could help

The term intermittent fasting has gained a great deal of traction over the last couple of years, both in popular culture and the scientific community. I often have patients ask me whether it could be helpful for them. There is mounting evidence to support its use in regulating blood sugar metabolism and in the treatment of obesity.

Intermittent fasting (IF) (or "digestive rest" as I like to call it) refers to the act of going longer periods of time without eating. To attain the metabolic benefits of digestive rest, the consensus appears to be a minimum fasting period of fourteen hours, while some people extend it to as much as eighteen hours. During that time, you are encouraged to stay hydrated and drink adequate amounts of water. It appears to be more beneficial to structure the eating window into the earlier part of the day, for example, 7:00 a.m.–5:00 p.m. Eating at night has been associated with increased rates of obesity and diabetes. This earlier-day eating window is also referred to as "circadian rhythm fasting." (There are also other methods of IF, where a person would spend two full days per week on a more restricted caloric intake, while eating their typical daily pattern the other five days. This is referred to as the 5:2 plan and is detailed by Kate Harrison in *The 5:2 Diet Book*.)

You may be wondering what effect this practice may have on your metabolism. Giving your digestive system an extended break appears to help reset some of the glucose and insulin signaling pathways, thereby improving insulin sensitivity. This has been studied in a controlled trial of patients with pre-diabetes, and lower insulin levels were documented in the group practicing digestive rest.

People with advanced diabetes and those on medications for diabetes, pregnant and breastfeeding women, and people with eating disorders should not attempt intermittent fasting unless under close supervision of their physician.

In my practice, I also extend the recommendation for digestive rest not only to patients who have dysregulated blood sugar and who are overweight, but also to patients who are having problems with digestive health. Extended periods of digestive rest have been shown to improve the health of the gut microbiome and reduce inflammation. There is also a growing body of research examining the effect of IF in cardiovascular disease, longevity, and even cancer.

The migratory motor complex (MMC)
Also called the migrating myoelectric complex, the MMC can be thought of as the innate process of sweeping the intestines between meals to push residual digestive debris down the digestive tract. It is characterized by a series of electrical-induced waves of smooth muscle contraction of the intestines. Secretions from the pancreas and stomach along with bile help with this cleansing process. The sounds of the MMC are characterized by growling and get shut off as soon as food is consumed. Interestingly, patients who have a motility disorder may have an observable absence of the MMC sounds in the fasted state. If you are constantly eating or tend to be a grazer, the MMC doesn't have much opportunity to operate and clear the intestines, which may result in imbalance of the gut flora and potentially inflammation.

What about leaky gut?
If you've done any amount of reading about gut health, you undoubtedly have come across the term leaky gut. This is referred to as "intestinal permeability" in the medical literature. There is a great deal of research that leaky gut can play a role in autoimmune disease. When lab testing indicates an increase in intestinal permeability, I first attempt to identify and treat the cause, which may include:

* SIBO

* microbiome imbalance

* infections

* diet, including food sensitivities

* medications

* stress

What is the best test for leaky gut?

Should you just assume you have it? When I am concerned about the presence of leaky gut, I recommend a zonulin test. It is a simple, relatively inexpensive test, only a $30 addon to the food sensitivity panel or to diagnostic stool testing that I order in my practice. Another test that can be used to assess intestinal permeability is a urine-based test that assesses absorption of lactulose.

What is malabsorption?

Malabsorption simply means there is a reduced capacity to absorb nutrients from the diet. Over time, this can create significant health problems from resultant nutrient deficiencies, such as anemia and osteoporosis. It's always important to determine the cause of malabsorption in order to correct the problem. Causes of malabsorption include infections, celiac disease, lactose intolerance and other enzyme deficiencies, inflammatory bowel disease, surgery that removes parts of the intestines, chronic use of laxatives and antibiotics, and damage from radiation treatments.

Are there tests for malabsorption?

The most common test to check for malabsorption is a fecal fat test where patients are asked to eat a higher fat diet for a few days while collecting stool samples. If too much fat is measured in the stool, it indicates that it's not being absorbed properly. Also from a stool testing panel, products of protein breakdown are often measured, and that can also indicate reduced ability to absorb protein. Other tests for malabsorption include the xylose absorption test and the lactulose/mannitol test.

Signs and symptoms of malabsorption

* food in stool
* foul-smelling and loose stool
* light colored stools
* stools that stick to the toilet bowl and are hard to flush away
* chronic diarrhea
* gas and burping
* bloating, abdominal distension
* weight loss
* scaly, dry skin

Advanced diagnostic stool testing

I covered this topic quite extensively in my book, *Unzip Your Genes*. These advanced panels are more widely available through functional laboratories across the United States. A comprehensive panel will include microbiome analysis using a technique called PCR, which measures DNA segments to determine the diversity and abundance of microbiome species in the intestinal tract, as well as checking for intestinal pathogens and parasites. Other important assessments on these panels include digestive function and biomarkers of intestinal inflammation.

CHAPTER 3

Eating

🔹 EATING VS. DIET—WHAT'S THE DIFFERENCE?

Diet is what you eat. Eating is an act. Eating is influenced by mood. How you feel can impact how you eat and what you eat. Some people are more affected by this more than others. As I detailed in the last chapter, bacteria in your gut can also trigger cravings and food-seeking behavior and even change mood. In Section 3, I will delve deeper into the impact of bitter emotions on your health, as that is a core element of my bitter prescription. It's a bitter pill to swallow to accept that these feelings may be sabotaging your health. In this chapter, I will focus on eating styles and behaviors.

🔹 EATING STYLE AND WHY IT MATTERS

We all have to eat. For most people, each day is filled with a series of choices of what to nourish their body with. It doesn't just matter what those foods actually are—the quality of those foods also matters, and the manner in which we eat matters (which I refer to as our "eating style"). When you first hear "eating style," you might think I'm talking about whether you eat a paleo or vegan diet, or practice intermittent fasting. Eating style involves attitude toward food, actual eating behavior, and relationship with food. If you've read my last book, *Unzip Your Genes*, you may remember that some of these behaviors are influenced by specific genes. For example, a behavior termed eating disinhibition is influenced by a genetic variation called a single nucleotide polymorphism (SNP). People affected by this gene can be more likely to overeat their favorite foods, have difficulty with portion control, and/or may be emotional eaters. This is just one example of an eating style.

The reason I am concerned about eating styles is that this is what tends to sabotage most people's healthy eating intentions. Most of the people who come to me want to follow a healthy diet, and the odd thing is that, when I review their diet, some of these people may already be eating a generally healthy diet, but their roadblock is actually their eating style.

A very interesting study about attitudes toward food was reported in the journal *Explore*. Researchers examined seven factors involved in eating and determined that certain eating styles were related to obesity and overeating. Many people just focus on what they eat, but patterns and attitudes toward eating. may be a contributing factor in whether they're able to stay in a healthy weight range.

Researchers developed questionnaires to measure food, nutrition, and eating themes in more than five thousand participants. The results helped the researchers identify seven eating styles that were independently related to overeating, and five that were significantly associated with people being overweight or obese. By analyzing the results of the questionnaires, researchers developed an integrative eating score, where those at the lowest end were the most obese. The eating styles of this group included: (1) emotional eating (2) consumption of more processed, fast, sweet, and fried foods and less fresh, whole grains, fruits, and vegetables (3) paying less attention to sensory and spiritual aspects of eating (4) focusing on self-judgment and feeling guilty about overeating (also called food fretting) (5) more likely eating in a hectic, tense atmosphere (6) more likely to eat while doing other things and (7) more likely eating by themselves.

Take a closer look at this list and identify whether any of your eating habits are similar.

Eating Styles Associated with Obesity
Emotional Eating (eating to manage feelings)
Fast Food (eating mostly processed, high-calorie food, less fresh food)
Food Fretting (judgmental thoughts and overconcern about food)
Task Snacking (eating while doing other activities)
Lack of Sensory, Spiritual Nourishment ("flavoring" food with meaning)
Eating Atmosphere (dining aesthetics and surroundings)
Social Fare (eating alone vs. with others)

This study shows that we should follow the wisdom of other cultures and the ways of the past: respect the world that provides us sustenance, express gratitude for nutritious, fresh food, appreciate the surroundings in which we eat, eat only when we are hungry, take time to prepare nutritious meals, and enjoy them in a relaxing atmosphere with the people we love, focusing on your meal and no other tasks.

The destructive habit of eating alone

We are the most advanced species on our planet, and we often skip the practice of sharing our meals together. Language is one of the main distinctions of being human. When we eat alone most of the time, we are acting like less evolved animals. The pleasure of sharing a meal with family, friends, or colleagues is good for our health. There is a reason there is a shared dining room in retirement homes, as it is known to improve the overall well-being of the residents.

➡ GENETIC TESTING AND EATING BEHAVIOR

In my book, *Unzip Your Genes*, I discussed six different gene variants that influence the relationship with food. I routinely order a genetic testing panel for my patients to discover which ones are sabotaging their best intentions. By being able to specifically target which eating behavior traits are at issue, a customized behavioral counseling plan can be developed to better address these issues. I covered these in my previous book, including the strategies that are most effective at addressing the behaviors.

The eating behavior traits are:

1. Eating disinhibition

2. Satiety

3. Food desire

4. Sweet tooth

5. Snacking

Eating disinhibition
In my practice, the most troublesome eating behavior that can be caused by a gene variant is eating disinhibition. It's quite common in people struggling to maintain a healthy weight. This is what can make some people more prone to emotional eating. When people with this gene are under more stress, they can be more likely to use food as a way to help them cope with it. I can't begin to count the number of patients who have been derailed by stress and turn to food as comfort.

Satiety

The issue of feeling satisfied or full after eating can be influenced by genetics. The FTO gene, also dubbed the "fat gene," can result in a sense of just never feeling full, so people tend to consume more calorie-rich foods in an attempt to satiate their appetite. Obviously, this increases the risk of obesity. One strategy to combat this problem is to consume foods that are likely to make you feel fuller. For example, when you eat an apple before dinner, you're more likely to feel full because the fiber in the apple (when accompanied by water) expands in your stomach. I prefer the use of bitter plants because they can delay emptying of the stomach, leading to a sense of feeling fuller more quickly without adding extra calories.

Food desire

Our general desire for food is extremely complex and influenced by a variety of factors. Genetics is one of those factors. There is a gene that influences how much effort someone is willing to exert to obtain a specific food. This SNP can impel you to change out of your pajamas, get into your car, and head off to the grocery store to get your favorite pint of ice cream or bag of potato chips. It's similar to those intense pregnancy cravings when women must have a particular food, no matter what time it is or how odd the craving.

Sweet tooth

While processed sugar tends to be highly addictive across the population, some people are particularly vulnerable to the risk of consuming higher amounts of sugar. There is a variant in a gene, that also predisposes to a higher risk of diabetes, that influences glucose sensing in the brain. This is referred to as the gene for sweet tooth.

Snacking

For obvious reasons, if we are continuously snacking or consuming high-calorie foods, then we end up gaining weight and eventually can become obese. The drive to snack can be influenced by your genetics. There is a gene that appears to impact two appetite-regulating hormones, leptin and chole-cystokinin (more on those later), resulting in more extreme snacking behavior.

In addition to the five eating behavior traits just reviewed, there are a few other factors that are very important to consider when reviewing eating patterns. One of these is another genetic factor that impacts how a person responds to changes in caloric intake from day to day, referred to as the weight loss and regain gene. The other factors to consider are how many calories are generally consumed on a regular basis, as well as the quality of the food consumed.

WEIGHT LOSS AND REGAIN

There is a genetic variant that makes it easier for you to regain weight after you have been on a lower-calorie diet. This gene is somewhat obvious to predict in people who notice that they can undo all their good dietary efforts in one indulgent meal or with the popularized "cheat day" that some fitness gurus recommend. The incidence of this gene in the population is quite common. If you are a carrier, it is important to consume a similar amount of food day to day, so your body knows what to expect on a regular basis. The key here is consistency.

Calories

As I said earlier, calories still matter if you need to lose weight from your midsection. Don't get caught up in trendy diets that tout unlimited calories. For example, there are ketogenic diet advocates claiming that calories don't matter and you can eat however much you want, as long as you keep your macros in balance and stay in a state of ketosis. This is simply not true if you need to shed excess belly fat.

⬤ FOOD QUALITY

As I already mentioned, the quality of our food supply matters. In addition to the lower levels of vitamins and minerals and the use of industrial chemicals, a major concern is lower phytonutrient content. This is a result of both factory farming and genetic modification of plants.

When plants are grown with chemical pesticides and fertilizers, they don't produce the same levels of bioactive compounds that serve the purpose of allowing the plant to thrive. These bioactive compounds are the very ones that impact the genetic potential of human DNA, referred to as epigenetic expression. Furthermore, these bioactive compounds tend to be bitter and can activate the bitter receptors, which I will cover more in depth in the next chapter.

The other condition that affects the quality of our diet is genetic modification of plants. Conventionally-grown plants have been bred over the years to contain less of these bioactive bitter-tasting compounds, with the intent that it would make that vegetable or fruit taste less bitter and enhance the sweet-ness to produce food that would match the changing palate of people accustomed to consuming the Standard American Diet, which is rich in sugar and processed food and stripped of their nutrients. Organically grown foods, by definition, cannot be genetically modified, so they will tend to have more bitter qualities. If you have access to heirloom varieties of produce through your local farmers' market or grocer, or you can obtain heirloom seeds to grow your own, even better, as these varieties tend to be rich in bitter bioactives.

CHAPTER 4

Bitters

➡ WHAT ARE BITTERS?

Up to this point, I have made brief references to bitters. Now, it's time to take a deeper dive into the history and science of bitters. The only exposure you may have had previously to the term *bitters* is as a cocktail ingredient. Those are indeed in the category of bitters, as they are an alcoholic preparation infused with botanical ingredients to intentionally impart a bitter flavor to drinks. Alcoholic bitters were very popular in the 1800s and were often served by aristocrats, as an apéritif, added to pre-dinner cocktails, or as a digestif, served after dinner to improve digestion. Alcoholic bitters have remained popular in Europe. In fact, on a recent trip when our family traveled to Spain, we visited Montserrat, a historic monastery built in 1025, where I had the opportunity to taste an alcoholic bitters blend made by monks who collected the herbs in the surrounding mountains to infuse into the beverage. Locals touted regular consumption of this bitter beverage as a way to keep them feeling younger. Alcoholic bitters are making a splash in the United States, gaining traction in recent years among the craft cocktail community. A favorite alcoholic bitter of mine is Campari, which is an Italian apéritif that can be used to make a variety of cocktails, such as Negronis, and is often mixed with Prosecco as a summer refresher in Italy.

Beyond alcoholic beverages, bitters are widely distributed in many other foods. Bitters are a category of biological compounds for which the tongue happens to have specialized taste receptors which register bitter taste in the brain. It was thought that bitter taste was simply an evolutionary protective mechanism to allow us to identify poisonous compounds (which are often bitter) in plants that were gathered or food that had spoiled. Bitter compounds in plants play an important role in plant survival by acting as a natural pesticide and deterrent to predators. Higher concentrations of bitter compounds are found in sprouts and seedlings, which makes sense as a protective mechanism for a small, vulnerable plant. (Pea sprouts are a hit with my kids, and I love the fact that these are more concentrated in bioactive compounds and vitamins.)

I am often in awe of the innate wisdom of nature to provide for us through plants that contain these unique compounds that not only gift us with the fuel to run our bodies, the vitamins and minerals that power all our complex biochemical reactions, but also the bitter bioactive compounds that can enhance our overall health. There are broad-reaching effects of bitters on the human body. We now know that there at least fifty different bitter taste receptors throughout the body that not only participate in our sensory system, but also play extremely important roles in digestion and metabolism. These bitter taste receptors can sense literally thousands of different bitter compounds.

Furthermore, these bitter taste receptors that bind bioactive compounds found in plants can have epigenetic effects, ultimately activating our DNA to help express optimal health potential. These bitter phytochemicals are known to play a role in prevention of a number of chronic diseases, including diabetes, cancer, and cardiovascular disease. Familiar examples of foods that contain bitters include kale, green tea, and lemons. In section two, we will delve deeper into dietary sources of bitters.

➡ BITTERS, GMOS, AND OUR HEALTH

Modern food production, and ultra-processing of foods, can strip the bitter compounds out of foods. Genetic modification of plants is an intentional way of changing the flavor profile to select for sweeter flavor and less bitter flavor. It is a well-known fact that the food industry removes phenols, flavonoids, isoflavones, terpenes, and glucosinolates from plant foods through selective breeding and a variety of debittering processes. Food chemists have taken the approach that these bitter phytonutrients are undesirable to the consumer palate and are therefore expendable. They come from the perspective that people spend more money on food for the taste, not the long-term health benefits. Debittering of the human diet is a massive public health problem. Bitter phytonutrients are involved in prevention of many chronic diseases. As consumers have become accustomed to the taste of non-bitter foods, as a direct result of the food industry, it poses a unique challenge for our society. I believe the solution will come through widespread education and spreading awareness of the problem we are facing, which is one of the intentions of this book.

As a culture, we are dealing with widespread obesity and skyrocketing rates of type 2 diabetes. I suspect part of the problem has been changing the balance of sweet and bitter compounds in our food supply, which can impact our cravings for sweets. When we consume more sweet-tasting compounds and less bitter ones, we end up craving more sweets. The occurrence of bitters in the diet is really important for the regulation of appetite. One way to get more bitters in your diet is to start growing and buying heirloom varieties of vegetables and fruits in an attempt to get closer to the dietary phytonutrient profile we consumed many years ago.

➡ Bitters in the Practice of Plant Medicine

Long before digestive aids such as enzymes and ox bile were used to support the function of the digestive system, bitter herbs were used by herbalists to enhance digestive function, especially in the elderly. Gentian (*Gentiana lutea*) is one the most well-known bitters that stimulates the production of hydrochloric acid in the stomach, as well as salivary, duodenal, and pancreatic digestive enzyme production. Obviously, if someone was dealing with too much acid production, then gentian would be an herb to avoid. Another example of the traditional herbal medicine application of bitters is with centaury (*Centaurium erythraea*), which is used to promote gastric secretions and improve bowel motility for someone with sluggish digestion. Probably the most commonly known bitter today is hops (Humulus lupulus), which most people recognize as a component of beer, but it's also used as a bitter plant medicine to aid digestion, especially for people who have a "nervous stomach," and can also help as a relaxant for trouble sleeping.

➡ The Bitter Taste Receptors

There are multiple taste receptors (type 2) that sense bitter compounds, referred to in the scientific literature as the TAS2Rs or T2Rs. When these receptors were first discovered, they were recognized as occurring only in the mouth, but later, they were found throughout the gastrointestinal tract: on the soft palate, nasopharynx, larynx, and esophagus, as well as into the intestine, in the airways, the kidneys, immune system, and even in the brain.

These receptors are so widely studied that there is even research now looking at the effects of genetic variation among these bitter taste receptors. There are also single nucleotide polymorphisms (SNPs) identified for the TAS2R receptors. For example, there is a specific dysfunctional TAS2R9 receptor that has been associated with increased risk of diabetes through affecting glucose and insulin signaling pathways. On the other hand, there is a genetic variant in the TAS2R16 gene that is associated with longevity, which was discovered in a study among people living in Southern Italy.

All bitter bioactives don't always register as bitter

Nature provides such a diverse group of chemical compounds, from amino acids to ureas and polyphenols, that many are seemingly unrelated other than their ability to bind bitter receptors. Although of many of the described compounds known to activate the bitter taste receptors actually taste bitter, oftentimes, these bitter biaoctives are not perceived in the brain as having a bitter taste. However, they still are affecting the downstream signaling cascade that is set off when the receptors are activated.

Bitter means it comes with bioactive

When you eat bitter-tasting plants, you know you are also getting a power-packed meal of bioactives. Bioactive compounds are defined as extra nutritional elements that are present in foods that are not considered essential to human health but have tremendous health benefits. Evolutionarily, tasting bitter was an important human quality when we foraged to determine whether plants were edible. The main class of compounds that activate the bitter taste receptors is the flavonoid group, which includes flavanones, flavonols, flavones, isoflavones, flavans (catechins), and anthocyanins. As I mentioned, these receptors can be activated without the perception of bitter taste. These chemical compounds are some of the most studied phytonutrients influencing human health. Other phenolic compounds and glucosinolates (which are found in high levels in cruciferous vegetables) also activate the bitter receptors.

➡ TASTER STATUS AND HOW GENETICS CAN INFLUENCE TASTE PERCEPTION

When taste testing is conducted in food science settings to determine the overall taste profile for a food product, participants are often asked to take a simple test to determine if they are a "supertaster," "taster" or a "non-taster." This is done through placing a small piece of paper that contains the bitter compound propylthiouracil (PROP). SNPs in the TAS2R38 gene influence the perception of bitter, and people who have more copies of the PAV-type SNPs tend to be more averse to the taste of bitter. The reason why this is important in taste testing situations is that bitter supertasters are also more sensitive to the taste for sweet and texture of fat. This is important in commercial food tasting, because perceived bitterness of foods is the primary reason a food is rejected and is a driver for food chemists to debitter foods. Interestingly, more women are found to be supertasters for bitter, and this is proposed to be linked ancestrally as protective mechanism to detect toxins. Bitter taste also tends to last longer in the mouth than taste for salty, sour, or sweet.

Number of bitter receptors varies and decreases with age

The total number of taste buds on the tongue varies widely among the population and greatly influences taste perception, including taste for bitter. By the time you turn fifty, the overall number of taste buds which contain the bitter taste receptors will be decreasing. On average, we start out with about ten thousand taste buds, but as we age, the number declines. Taste buds have the ability to regenerate and turn over every couple weeks. This explains why we can regain taste in a just a few days after the tongue is damaged by consuming a hot beverage or food.

Perception of bitter is not just genetic, it's also affected by diet

There are more than fifty genes that code for bitter taste receptors, and we know that genetics definitely affects your bitter sensing system. However, your current diet can also affect how bitter foods taste. First of all, bitter taste is affected by the types of naturally occurring bacteria in the mouth, which is largely the result of current dietary habits. Second, proteins found in saliva influence taste perception, and the composition of diet determines which proteins make up saliva. If you are not eating a broad range of vegetables and bitter plants, when you initially start eating these, they may taste unpleasant. The good news is that over time, as they become a regular part of your diet, the proteins in your saliva change in a way that makes these foods taste more appealing to you and less bitter. As long as you are eating bitter compounds in your diet, no matter if they taste bitter or not, they will bind to the bitter taste receptors that set off the cascade of beneficial metabolic effects.

THE ROLE OF BITTERS IN HUMAN HEALTH

We are learning more about the role of bitter compounds and how they interact with receptors throughout the body. This is an area of study that has become very active. Well established is the fact that dietary bitter compounds activating these receptors is important for overall digestive function, lowering overall food intake and limiting blood sugar spikes after eating. The great news about bitters is that they can help regulate appetite, improve the digestive process, help with weight loss, and crush cravings for sweets. They also appear to play a role in such diverse activities as blood pressure regulation, thyroid function, and even brain health.

Bitters, oxidative stress, and chronic disease

In the first chapter, I discussed the role of inflammation and oxidative stress in the development of most chronic diseases associated with aging. This is really where bitter bioactive compounds in food play a starring role in human health and the prevention of chronic disease. These compounds not only act as direct antioxidants, but they also have the ability to induce our built-in (endogenous) antioxidant system and reduce inflammatory mediators. Some bitter compounds, like glucosinolates, also protect us against carcinogenic chemicals. Lower rates of colon cancer have been observed in people who consume higher amounts of green leafy vegetables and cabbage.

Bitters improve the digestive process

While bitter taste receptors in the mouth appear to be primarily involved in the perception of bitter compounds, bitter receptors lower down in the intestinal tract are thought to play a larger role in regulating digestion and metabolism. These receptors are involved in motility in the intestinal tract as well as maintaining blood sugar balance. Improved digestion is one of the first things people notice when they increase the amount of bitters in the diet, especially in my clinic when I recommend a potent nutritional supplement containing bitter medicinal plants.

Bitters help regulate appetite

Since the discovery that there are many different genetic variants of bitter taste receptors, researchers have been detailing relationships of receptor profiles in different people and their related dietary intake. There are trends showing genetic sensitivity to bitter taste and avoidance of the intake of bitter compounds found in healthy vegetables, which can be associated with more carbohydrate intake and being overweight. However, the research is complex here, because in other studies, female non-tasters have also been shown to trend toward obesity.

More importantly, when bitter receptors in the gut are activated by eating bitter foods, hormones related to appetite and satiety, like leptin and adiponectin, are triggered. Bottom line here is that, even though some people may find bitter foods aversive and tend to avoid them, they should really push themselves to consume more bitter compounds to gain the health benefits. As I mentioned, when you eat more bitter foods, over time the composition of proteins in the saliva changes in a way that makes those foods taste more pleasant.

Bitters, intestinal hormones, and blood sugar balance
The lesser-known intestinal hormones referred to as gut-derived hormones are extremely important in regulating blood sugar metabolism and appetite. These are:

* ghrelin
* cholecystokinin (CCK)
* glucose-dependent insulinotropic polypeptide (GIP)
* glucagon-like peptide-1 (GLP-1)
* peptide YY (PYY).

Ghrelin is released in a fasting state, and it can drive you to seek food, while the other four hormones, CCK, GIP, GLP-1, and PYY, are released after you eat and reduce further food seeking—in other words, they make you feel satiated. Bitter dietary compounds activate the bitter receptors, which modulate these gut hormones in a favorable pattern leading to both reductions in blood glucose and appetite.

Bitter compounds such as resveratrol, which is found in higher concentrations in red wine, can improve insulin sensitivity, even in diabetics, which thereby can improve blood sugar control. There are many other bitter components, including EGCG (green tea) and berberine, that have been widely observed to help regulate glucose levels.

I remember first hearing about bitter melon about twenty years ago when I was a medical student and learned how this fruit was traditionally used in Asian cultures as medicine. The scientific name for bitter melon is *Momordica charantia* and is also commonly called bitter gourd, karela, or balsam pea. It can help regulate insulin levels, address obesity, inflammation, oxidative stress, and even help with infections. This fruit tastes extremely bitter, but there are plenty of traditional Chinese recipes for meals that include bitter melon.

Bitters, obesity, and weight loss

Consumption of bitter compounds can delay stomach emptying, leading to a sense of feeling full more quickly. As a result, bitters can reduce the number of calories consumed, and that alone, could help reduce rates of obesity and help shed excess pounds. But bitters do far more for us than just helping us feel full. Bitter compounds affect so many parts of our digestive function: everything from enhancing all phases of digestive function, regulating hormones that control appetite, improving glucose control and insulin sensitivity, reducing intestinal inflammation (a known cause of obesity), and even improving microbiome health (which we know can also impact our appetite and metabolism).

Crush cravings for sweets with bitters

A relatively common complaint that patients bring up to me is that they have intense cravings for sweets. Oftentimes, it hits them mid-afternoon, and they describe being compelled to satisfy that desire for sweet. They know they really should stop eating sweets but find it hard to stop. Like any addiction, sugar cravings are subject to the same extreme difficulty of merely exerting willpower. Sugar cravings are complex, but the taste receptors do play a role here.

The dietary plan I have found to be very helpful for people with sugar cravings is the Bitter Prescription (found in section two of this book). I often start them with a more intensive "bitter pill" which is a blend of bitter herbs that they take prior to meals. Not only does this tend to reduce their cravings for sweets more quickly, it can also improve all aspects of their digestion and metabolism. Over time, eating a diet rich in bitter bioactives can take away those cravings completely.

Bitters and the microbiome

The health of the bacteria in the gut has been tied to body composition. Specifically, lower levels of *Bacteroidetes* and higher amounts of *Firmicutes* in the large intestine has been observed in obese populations. Consumption of a broad range of bitter dietary compounds positively impacts the health of the gut microbiome and can shift the balance toward higher levels of *Bacteroidetes*. Some data indicates that the types of bacteria in the gut influence both the number and types of taste receptors found in the body, which can influence food-seeking behavior. Bacteria that live in your mouth can impact your taste perception for bitters.

Bitters and immune health

Many bitter plant compounds are potent antimicrobials against pathogenic bacteria, viruses, and yeast. In my clinical practice, we use bitter plant medicines routinely as very effective ways to combat a wide variety of infections. Interestingly, research has shown that resveratrol applied topically to sores caused by the herpes simplex virus could reduce the rate of viral spread and could even be used to treat cold sores at first sign of an outbreak. Besides acting as direct antibiotics, bitter compounds can impact our immune system in a variety of ways. Bitters can support a chronically stressed immune system for people who are prone to recurrent infections and/or don't recover quickly from them, as well as immune systems that have switched to an autoimmune response, with curcumin (found in turmeric) sitting at the top of the list.

Bitters and cardiovascular health

One of the main classes of bitter compounds, referred to as flavonoids, are well known to protect against oxidation of LDL cholesterol, thereby interrupting an important part of the development of atherosclerotic plaque. By reducing the available free radicals in the body, there are then less reactive oxygen species to damage LDL particles. In fact, people who consume higher amounts of flavonoids in the diet have been shown to have lower rates of coronary heart disease. Of important note is the finding that there are bitter taste receptors found on the heart muscle and the large blood vessels leading out of the heart. These receptors are thought to be important in regulating the strength of the contractions of the heart. Research has shown that stimulation of these bitter receptors can improve blood pressure control. Also interesting is the finding that the heart can increase expression of bitter taste receptors when it is failing, which is proposed to be a protective mechanism to slow down the rate of decline. There is certainly a lot more to learn about the role of bitter receptors in heart health.

Bitters and bone health

Bone loss associated with aging, referred to as osteopenia if it is mild and osteoporosis if it is more severe, is a major concern for many of my patients. Malabsorption of nutrients and low stomach acid are risk factors for increased rates of bone loss. Chronic inflammation is one of the major underlying factors in osteoporosis. Bitter dietary compounds can help reduce inflammation, improve digestive function, and enhance absorption of nutrients.

Bitters and brain health

You may remember that I mentioned bitter receptors are also found in the brain. I always say, if there are receptors found somewhere, they serve some purpose. Previous research has shown that the bitter-tasting iso-alpha acids (IAAs) in the hops plant (commonly used in beer) can help prevent brain inflammation and Alzheimer's pathologies in mice. Lower risk of developing neurodegenerative diseases has been observed in people who drink low-to-moderate levels of alcoholic beverages daily versus those who abstain from alcoholic beverages or drink excessively. Researchers believe this is partly due to the effects of alcohol itself, along with compounds that activate the bitter receptors like the IAAs in beer and resveratrol in wine. Bitter compounds can possibly delay memory problems associated with aging though multiple mechanisms including affecting blood flow to the brain, enzymes associated with aging, and inflammatory mediators.

⬤ BITTERS AND MOOD

I find this association completely fascinating, because in deciding on a title for this book, I had wanted to make sure that I was able to tie together emotional health with nutrition. In the reception area of my clinic, there is a popular book that many of my patients browse while they are waiting for their appointment. The book is *The Kitchen Shrink* by Natalie Savona. It describes how these bioactive compounds impact our mood and can boost our mental capacity. Bitter compounds like resveratrol, quercetin, and proanthocyanidins can help regulate neurotransmitters that impact mood, such as serotonin, dopamine, and noradrenaline.

CHAPTER 5

Hormonal Balance

The goal of this chapter is to gain a better understanding of hormones, and how diet and emotions affect them. I will also discuss the role of good quality sleep in maintaining good health as you age. As you may have already experienced, sleeping problems become much more common after you turn thirty-five. If you are female and have passed that age and have not yet experienced an unrestful night, you are lucky! It is a terrible feeling to wake up and have trouble falling back to sleep. Women are twice as likely as men to have trouble falling asleep or staying asleep.

In my clinical practice, two of the more common issues I see affecting people as they age are sleep disturbances and stress. For that reason, I will devote an uneven amount of content to these two topics, because they are some of the most impactful issues affecting our overall health. I will also review hormones related to aging, digestion, fat metabolism, and appetite, because these don't get as much attention as the sex hormones (estrogen, progesterone, and testosterone) and thyroid hormone. First, let's talk about sleep.

➡ SLEEP

I always tell patients that, without good sleep, healing is difficult. This is why, when a patient tells me that they are having a problem sleeping, it will be one of my top priorities to address right away, before we start working on anything else. People who don't get enough sleep tend to have an increased appetite, experience trouble with satiety, and can eat more calories during the day, resulting in weight gain. Sleep issues can be caused by some other medical conditions, so you should see your physician to rule out medical causes like an overactive thyroid (hyperthyroidism or Graves' disease). Chronic pain is a common cause of both sleep disruption and poor sleep quality. Difficulty sleeping can also be a manifestation of a mood disorder.

Getting good quality sleep is very important for healthy cortisol balance, but unfortunately, that is easier said than done for many people. I routinely treat patients for insomnia, which can present in different ways. Some people have difficulty falling asleep, which is referred to as sleep latency, while others may have trouble staying asleep or suffer from frequent waking. Even worse is the duo, "Can't get to sleep or stay asleep." Patients also describe non-restful sleep, where they feel tired when they wake up in the morning after a full night of sleep. Also, people can experience poor sleep quality and don't even know it until they start using a biometric device, such as a Fitbit, to measure the patterns of deep sleep.

What is a good amount of sleep?
I am asked this question often, and it really is a range of about seven to eight hours per night. I am also concerned about the quality of that period of sleep, meaning how much is deep, restorative sleep. In general, women tend to need a little more sleep than men. Too much sleep and too little sleep have both been linked to poor health outcomes.

What happens during sleep cycles?
Not as much is known about REM, the dream state, as is known about deep sleep, in which growth hormone is released and repair and regeneration of tissues occurs. We do know that, as

we age, we get less deep sleep, and this is thought to speed up the aging process. When we sleep, we sleep in a series of four to six cycles that proceeds through light to deep, back to light, and then into REM:

N1–N2–N3–N2–N1–REM

Each stage has unique characteristics and carries an ideal range summarized in this table:

Stages of sleep	Level of Sleep	Ideal range/ night	Effects
N1	Very Light	5%	Just falling asleep
N2	Light	50%	Transitioning to deep sleep, metabolism regulation
N3	Deep	25%	HGH released, repair and regeneration
REM	Dream state	20%	Shallow breath, high brain activity, limb paralysis

➥ WHAT AFFECTS SLEEP CYCLES?

There are many lifestyle factors that can affect sleep cycles. When I am assessing a patient with insomnia, I am first looking for these main factors to see if there is anything we can remove or add that could help with their sleep or that simply helps us explain what might be causing the sleep problem, such as aging. I divide these into two simple categories:

Good for sleep

* Magnesium intake

* Exercise

* Meditation

Bad for sleep

* Shift work/timing of sleep

* Eating certain types of food or meals close to bedtime

* Aging

* Caffeine

* Medications: antidepressants (can completely suppress REM), decongestants

* Nicotine

* Alcohol

SLEEP HYGIENE

After assessing these lifestyle factors, then I look at what is referred to as sleep hygiene (a behavioral approach to sleep medicine that was developed in the 1970s) to determine if there are simple changes that could be made to help improve sleep quality.

* Same time to bed

* Natural light exposure

* Napping during the day

* Dark room

* No blue light two hours before bed

* Comfortable bedding, mattress, and pillow

* Cold room. Not too many covers

If all of these factors are addressed and the person is still having problems with sleep, then I consider adrenal function and/or the short-term use of medicinal plants and nutritional supplements like L-theanine and GABA to get the sleep cycle back on track.

➥ WHAT IS CORTISOL?

Cortisol is a steroid hormone secreted by the adrenal glands. These vital glands sit just above the kidneys and are responsible for many critical aspects of metabolism. The adrenal glands also secrete DHEA, aldosterone, adrenaline, and noradrenaline. Cortisol is involved in blood sugar control, immune function, inflammation, blood pressure, memory, water and salt balance, and even plays a role in pregnancy. Cortisol secretion from the adrenal glands is stimulated by both emotional and physical stress, excessive exercise, and perceived low blood sugar levels (referred to as hypoglycemia). In rare cases, excess cortisol can be caused by a serious medical condition like an adrenal tumor, so, again, I would emphasize making sure you have been worked up by a physician.

Why are high levels of cortisol so bad?
At the deepest level, cortisol changes the expression of your genes. Cortisol directly affects DNA methylation patterns, resulting in a cascade of effects in many different systems. Cortisol also contributes to the deposition of belly fat. Blood sugar levels can elevate in response to cortisol secretion. Elevated cortisol (and chronic stress) speeds up the aging process, and who wants that?

Is there a test for cortisol?
There are a number of ways to assess cortisol levels. It is relatively easy to screen cortisol using blood testing, typically

with a fasting morning sample. The problem with this method is if that, if at this one time point, it happens to be normal, you are missing the rest of the day. Cortisol levels fluctuate throughout the day and can spike out of normal range. There is also a twenty-four-hour urinary cortisol test, but that can also provide false negatives, because at some points, your cortisol levels may be borderline low, while other time points cortisol may be elevated, so it can get canceled out on a total cortisol test. My favorite test is the four time-point salivary test, which captures a better picture of the pattern of cortisol secretion throughout the day.

What is cortisol resistance?

As a result of chronic stress, the hypothalamic-pituitary-adrenal (HPA) axis can become disordered, and people can experience a loss of the circadian rhythm of cortisol production. The normal pituitary and hypothalamic responses to cortisol are not turned off, as is normally the case in a negative feedback loop, because the receptors for cortisol have become resistant. Receptor resistance can occur with insulin and leptin, too. When we measure four-point salivary cortisol, if the pattern changes to a flat line instead of the typical circadian ebb and flow, it indicates cortisol resistance. This can have profound effects on the immune system. Fortunately, the circadian rhythm can be reset, but in order to do so, good quality sleep habits must be present. Through the use of adaptogenic herbs, the negative feedback loop of the HPA is increased, and cortisol balance can be re-established.

Exercise and cortisol

Physical activity level is a bit of a double-edged sword when it comes to managing cortisol levels. Some people report that intense exercise is critical for managing the stress in their life, but exercise that is very strenuous actually induces a rise in cortisol in the short term. Mild to moderate exercise has been shown to result in lower cortisol levels at night.

Bitter feelings, mindset, and cortisol

One of the most powerful ways to control cortisol is to manage how you react to the stressors in your life. The brain perceives emotional stress the same way as an actual external threat, mounting the stress response as if there were an internal metabolic or physical stress. Even social isolation, which is increasingly common in our digital age, is a perceived stressor. The adrenal glands are responsible for the fight-or-flight response, and your perception of your environment sets off a cascade of biochemical responses. Bitter feelings, like irritability, chronic worry, and fear, even at a low level, can affect adrenal secretion of hormones. While many times, it is difficult to control your environment and the actual stressors you are exposed to (although, this is an entire topic on its own, because, oftentimes, many of our stressors are self-inflicted), you can learn to control your responses. There are many effective techniques to become less reactive to stressors and perceived stress, with meditation arguably being the best.

Meditation and yoga practice

Meditation promotes a state of calmness and allows those who practice it to become more responsive in a productive way when reacting to a particular situation. Very basic anatomy of brain function explains this process. The neural connections among centers in the brain that control fear and anxiety and the ego are altered in a positive way in people who regularly meditate. In order to maintain these pathways, you must meditate on a regular basis. We also understand that vagal tone is associated with improved capacity to regulate stress responses and can be influenced by breathing patterns practiced in meditation and yoga.

Stress resiliency

Two people exposed to same stressor will not have the same outcome, which has been well documented in the setting of people exposed to military conflicts and victims of trauma. This also plays out in all of us with the routine daily stress of living in our fast-paced modern society. A genomic test panel that I order on many of my patients analyzes genes related to stress resiliency and helps explain why some people can tolerate higher levels of stress. If you are affected by this gene, the practice of meditation and yoga, as explained in the last paragraph, can positively contribute to stress resilience and even the mitigation of depression and anxiety symptoms.

Supplements that affect cortisol

There are many nutritional and herbal supplements that affect cortisol, but I do have my favorites that I use in my clinical practice. The class of herbal medicines that are used to improve homeostasis, or balance, of the HPA axis is referred to as adaptogens. These botanical medicines have been a mainstay in my therapeutic approach to regulating the stress response for the last twenty years. Nutritional supplements also provide foundational support for balanced adrenal function.

Techniques to help lower cortisol
Deep breathing
Yoga
Guided imagery
Meditation
Quality sleep

► ADAPTOGENS

Adaptogens are defined simply as plant medicines that increase the ability of the body to cope with stress. There are specific criteria that determine whether an herb can be classified as an adaptogen. It must be non-toxic and relatively free of adverse effects. And it must also act in both a nonspecific manner to improve resiliency to stress and possess a normalizing effect, whereby it brings the function back into balance from over-function (hyper) or under-function (hypo). Adaptogens have broad reaching effects on the endocrine, nervous, cardiovascular, and immune system. We know that adaptogens can reduce inflammation through modulation of immune function, which can even impact mood disorders. Some of my favorite adaptogenic plant medicines include ashwagandha (*Withania somnifera*), eleuthero (*Eleutherococcus senticosus*), rhodiola (*Rhodiola rosea*), and licorice (*Glycyrrhiza glabra*). Based on the unique clinical picture of each patient, I would select which plant medicines are the best fit.

► NUTRITIONAL THERAPY

Bodies under chronic stress have higher demands for certain vitamins and nutritional factors. Supplementation with fish oil has been shown to prevent activation of adrenals in people under emotional stress. Fish oil has long been recommended by naturopathic doctors as a nourishing supplement to support healthy adrenal function. Vitamin C and B vitamins, especially vitamins B2, B5, and B6, are helpful at supporting cellular energy, neurotransmitter, and catecholamine production. Phosphatidylserine can help normalize cortisol levels. Magnesium loss from the body is increased under higher levels of stress. This is a big issue, because dietary sources of magnesium are lower than ever due to depletion of the soil, so many people are at risk for deficiency.

➡ DO DIETARY PATTERNS AFFECT CORTISOL?

The short answer is yes. People who have issues with regulating blood sugar levels can also have problems with cortisol. When the body perceives too drastic a drop in blood sugar level (and this could technically still be within the normal range), cortisol is released to get the blood sugar levels back up to "normal." This can even happen during the night while sleeping, resulting in waking but not necessarily feeling hungry. This issue should be addressed with a health care provider trained in nutritional therapy who can work on personalized meal planning to help improve blood sugar control. Intermittent fasting, or digestive rest can help regulate blood sugar levels.

Foods that can help lower cortisol
Green and black tea
Dark chocolate
Water—avoid dehydration
Fermented foods

➡ DHEA

Dehydroepiandrosterone is an androgenic hormone released mostly from the adrenal glands. It is a complex hormone that effects many different systems in the body including skin, immune, musculoskeletal, and nervous system. It is a precursor for estrogen and testosterone. When I am assessing adrenal function in my patients, I routinely order a DHEA-sulfate test, which better reflects the body's reserves of DHEA. As we age, DHEA levels naturally decline, but excessive emotional and physical stress can lower DHEA levels. DHEA plays a role in fat metabolism, especially in limiting storage of belly fat and maintaining muscle mass, and it has been proposed as a treatment for obesity for people who have documented low levels of DHEA. DHEA supplementation should only be considered upon consultation with a physician if testing demonstrates deficiency, and levels must be monitored regularly. There are contraindications for DHEA supplementation, including hormone-sensitive cancers such as breast, prostate and adenomas, polycystic ovarian syndrome (PCOS), and prostate enlargement.

➡ PREGNENOLONE

Another precursor hormone, pregnenolone, is made inside many cell types throughout the body, including adrenal cells. Pregnenolone is the precursor of DHEA and, similarly, decreases with age. Lower production can also occur in people who are not getting enough sleep, exercising excessively, taking statin medications, are malnourished, and in hypothyroidism. The same cautions apply to pregnenolone as DHEA. People who have epilepsy, meningiomas, or take medications that affect GABA levels shouldn't take it. Again, you should work with a physician if you are considering hormone supplementation and have your levels monitored regularly.

➡ MELATONIN

Many people associate melatonin only with sleep, but it is also known as an anti-stress hormone, as it can oppose cortisol. It also regulates immunity and some aspects of the aging process, including growth hormone production (more on that next). Melatonin is a potent antioxidant and can protect cells from DNA damage. Excessive mental stress, poor sleeping habits, inadequate darkness throughout the night, insufficient exposure to natural light during daytime hours, and drinking too many caffeinated or alcoholic beverages close to bedtime can decrease melatonin production. This is another hormone that decreases as we age, and levels are down about 50 percent by the time we turn sixty. Make no wonder, we can have trouble sleeping as we get older. Recent research has shown that melatonin supplementation can reduce inflammatory markers and may even improve weight loss. Interestingly, melatonin can also be found in red wine. Now, I would not suggest a glass of red wine before bed to help with sleep, because the alcohol in there can dysregulate the sleep cycle. Because melatonin is a hormone, you should discuss supplementation with your doctor, because there are conditions where people should not take melatonin, such as certain immune system cancers, like lymphoma and leukemia, autoimmune diseases, and with some medications.

GROWTH HORMONE (GH)

Produced in the pituitary gland, growth hormone (also referred to as somatotropin and HGH, for human growth hormone) declines dramatically as we get older. At about age twenty-one, levels start to decline by about 15 percent per decade, and by the time we are sixty years old, our growth hormone levels will have dropped by more than 50 percent. Growth hormone secretion is inhibited by another hormone in our bodies called somatostatin, which increases as we age.

As you may have assumed, growth hormone is responsible for growth when we are young, but also continues to help with cellular growth and regeneration in our adult years. This hormone is produced in pulses while we are in the deep stages of sleep. GH is responsible for growing taller, and it's interesting when parents report colloquially that their teenager must have grown inches taller overnight!

What symptoms are reported to be associated with low GH?
There are many symptoms that have been attributed to declining levels of growth hormone. At the top of the list sits weight gain, loss of muscle mass with an increase in body fat, low energy, and mood swings. Although there is the potential for adverse effects, HGH injectables are available by prescription only, and in clinics where this treatment is used, patients often report noticing some of the following effects:

* improved exercise tolerance and overall strength

* more energy

* improved skin texture and elasticity

* balanced mood

* change in body composition—fat loss and muscle gain

* better sleep quality

* sharper memory and cognitive ability

Natural ways to improve GH function
Injectable HGH therapy is very expensive and not without risk. Furthermore, it is absolutely contraindicated in certain medical histories or illnesses. Safer approaches to boost GH activity in the body are some of the very methods that I recommend in this book, including:

* reducing excess belly fat

* digestive rest (intermittent fasting), especially limiting food intake in the evening

* limiting overall intake of simple sugars and improving insulin resistance

* getting optimal sleep

* exercise

➡ ADIPONECTIN

Adiponectin is the most abundant hormone released from fat cells. Its primary role is in the regulation of glucose and fat metabolism, but it is also a natural anti-inflammatory. Having low levels of adiponectin is associated with increased rates of obesity, insulin resistance, type 2 diabetes, and metabolic syndrome. Adiponectin also positively impacts cardiovascular function, reduces the propensity to build plaque in the arteries, improves insulin sensitivity, and reduces inflammation. High adiponectin levels are associated with reduced risk for type 2 diabetes. There are genetic factors that make people more prone to low adiponectin. Adiponectin can be measured through a simple blood test.

Factors that may improve adiponectin levels

Insulin-sensitizing, anti-diabetic drugs given to insulin-resistant type 2 diabetics can cause an increase in adiponectin levels. Other ways to increase adiponectin naturally are:

* caloric restriction
* weight loss
* fish oil supplementation

➡ LEPTIN

Leptin is a metabolic hormone that signals the brain that enough fat has been stored, to decrease caloric intake and burn calories at a normal rate. Leptin is found in the fat tissue, blood vessels, stomach, and even the placenta. The receptors that bind leptin are found in these same places but also in a part of the brain called the hypothalamus. Leptin crosses the blood-brain barrier to get to the brain, where it is thought to exert its main effect on behavior in lowering food intake. As you age, leptin activity gets blocked in the brain through the effects of ghrelin.

Leptin resistance

Having high levels of leptin has a similar effect to having high levels of circulating insulin. Similar to insulin resistance, you can also become resistant to the effects of leptin. Leptin resistance can occur in response to overeating, higher levels of glucose, body mass index, percentage of body fat, and alcohol intake. Not only is leptin involved in appetite, metabolic rate, and fat metabolism, it has also been implicated in a number of health problems beyond obesity. For example, leptin plays a role in pain pathways, and reduced levels of leptin are equated to lower levels of pain. Also, leptin has been implicated in autoimmune disease.

Addressing leptin resistance

The goal with leptin is to improve long-term control, thereby improving leptin sensitivity. Leptin balance is important. Too little or too much leptin perception are both problematic. Deficiency of leptin has been documented in severely obese children. If the brain is perceiving low leptin levels, then it will trigger us to eat more. Not getting enough sleep has been associated with increased caloric intake the next day, and it is quite likely that this is the result of the leptin pathway. Ways to improve leptin sensitivity include:

* improving sleep quality
* regular exercise
* diet lower in saturated fat and higher in mono-unsaturated fats (like olive oil)
* green tea
* curcumin
* omega-3 fatty acids like fish oil

➥ GHRELIN

Ghrelin is a fast-acting hormone in the stomach that exerts its action through the vagus nerve. It is referred to as the hunger hormone, because it signals us to eat when we have an empty stomach, but it also plays roles in regulating glucose and energy balance, cardioprotection, muscle atrophy, bone metabolism, and cancer. As I mentioned, ghrelin is also thought to inhibit leptin's action in the hypothalamus.

➥ INSULIN

When you eat, insulin is released by the pancreas to allow glucose to get inside your cells. Insulin is critical. If you have an insulin-dependent diabetic in your life, you are well aware of how important this hormone is. Type 1 diabetes is a life-threatening autoimmune disorder that destroys the islet cells in the pancreas which produce insulin, requiring injectable insulin to stay alive. There is a very strong genetic component in type 1 diabetes, and once the disease develops, it is irreversible. Damage to the pancreas from trauma, or other diseases, can also cause someone to become entirely dependent on insulin.

On the other hand, type 2 diabetes has a completely different origin and is a separate metabolic problem. It is the result of a specific pattern of long-term dietary habits, eating too much carbohydrate in the diet, causing the insulin receptors on cells to become resistant to its effects (termed insulin resistance). Glucose levels rise in the bloodstream, because it can't enter cells as well. Several genes can make some people more prone to developing type 2 diabetes, but some can be "turned off" with a Mediterranean diet. Type 2 diabetes is preventable, and even reversible in the earlier stages with therapeutic lifestyle changes, including diet and exercise.

● GERANYLGERANIOL (GG)

Most people have never heard of GG and for good reason, because this naturally occurring biochemical (which is not a hormone but does impact progesterone and testosterone levels) only became understood in the last decade. GG declines with aging. It is critical for making new proteins in the body (necessary for maintaining lean body mass), CoQ10 and vitamin K. GG also plays diverse roles in bodily function including pain control, inflammation, bone density, brain health, and even in cancer.

SECTION 2

The Bitter Prescription Dietary Plan

*T*his is not a crash diet, a fad diet, or the latest craze. It's straight-up real food based on traditional eating patterns around the world. This is a food plan for life. It should not leave you feeling deprived. You should only continue to feel better as this style of eating becomes your way of life. Can you drink coffee and tea? Yes. Can you drink wine? Yes. Do you have to prepare separate meals for yourself and your family? No. Can you eat in a restaurant? Yes. In fact, here's what it may look like. You order a cup of warm water with lemon first. You order a green salad dressed with oil and vinegar. Your entree is grilled chicken with a fresh, mixed vegetable medley. And, you have eaten a balanced breakfast and lunch, too. Sounds normal, right? You've probably eaten similar meals many times in the past (probably not with the lemon water, though).

So, what's the catch? The catch is what you include in those meals, specifically, a diverse array of colorful vegetables, prepared with herbs and spices that are packed with health-promoting phytochemicals that I refer to as bitter bioactives. And, starting the meal with bitters—the lemon, the green salad (choose arugula or watercress when you can)—helps stimulate better digestive function.

What is not part of the actual meal, and what is critical for overall health, is how well nutrients are digested and absorbed, and the health of the microbiome. The foods outlined in this plan can improve digestive health by stimulating better digestive function and balancing gut bacteria. If your digestive system needs some more intensive support, you may need to employ some additional nutritional therapy strategies (some of which I referred to in the first section) and should consider seeing a naturopathic physician or similarly trained licensed medical provider who specializes in nutrition.

I really hope you took the time to read the first section of this book, but if you are like a bunch of people I know, you just jumped ahead to see what my plan is all about. So, I encourage you to stop now and go back and read the first section to get the best results from this book. And for the rest of you, now we get into the nitty gritty and learn all about the Bitter Prescription dietary plan. The first chapter is about fat loss. I really want to emphasize that this section is for people who are retaining excess stored body fat. *If you are dealing with disordered eating and are underweight, I urge you to skip this chapter completely and pick up in Chapter 7: Bitter Prescription Dietary Essentials.*

CHAPTER 6

Fat Loss

SETTING A FAT LOSS GOAL

The rates of obesity have skyrocketed, and while there are people who are maintaining optimal body composition, in my clinical experience, most people who come to see me are not in that healthy zone. In section 1, I discussed why a healthy level of fat stores is so important and how carrying excess fat stores is a cause of chronic inflammation. This sets you up for premature aging and higher risk of chronic diseases. Knowing where you are, and where you should be, to reduce your risk and slow down the aging process is the first step to fat loss. Like any other area in life, to be successful you need to get clear on where you are now and where you need to go. Simply put, without setting goals, most people do not succeed. Committing to lifestyle changes can be challenging, and these simple measures can improve the chances of success.

USING TECHNOLOGY TO GUIDE FAT LOSS

In my practice, we use body composition testing. This is a machine that allows us to assess fat mass and muscle mass. It provides a more complete picture than just measuring weight on the scale, which doesn't tell us anything about how much lean body mass, fat, and water is contributing to that number. Knowing your numbers is very important. For example, I routinely see women who are within the normal range of BMI (body mass index), but their fat mass is too high, and their lean mass (made up mostly of muscle and bone) is too low. BMI is the calculation used to assess whether a person is underweight, overweight, obese, or morbidly obese. Body composition devices can be found in some doctor's offices and fitness centers. The device we use in our clinic is called an InBody, and it shows us the exact number of pounds of fat loss (and/or muscle gain) needed to reach optimal range. This makes it easier to develop a fat loss target for our patients at the same time we are designing their nutrition plan.

➡ HOW TO CALCULATE TARGET WEIGHT WITHOUT A MEDICAL DEVICE

If you don't have access to a body composition machine, then you can use a BMI calculation to determine what your healthy weight should be. As I said, BMI is not the best way to assess whether you have excess fat stores. The BMI calculation is limited if you have a low muscle mass, as I just described, and are in the healthy range. Also, if you have a very high muscle mass, then your BMI calculation may actually put you in an overweight category, which doesn't reflect your true risk status related to how much fat mass you have stored. Waist circumference is another method to determine if you have elevated risk due to excess belly fat. Risk elevates for women with a waist circumference over thirty-five inches, while for men, the cutoff is forty inches.

Calculating BMI (Body Mass Index)

There are BMI calculators widely available online, and that is really the simplest way to calculate your BMI. The standard BMI calculator on the National Institutes of Health website is a great resource.

* Underweight: under 18.5 kg/m^2
* Normal weight: 18.5-24.9 kg/m^2
* Overweight: 25-29.9 kg/m^2
* Obese: 30 kg/m^2
* Morbid obesity: above 35 kg/m^2 and experiencing obesity-related health conditions like diabetes or high blood pressure, *or* above 40 kg/m^2

SETTING CHECKPOINTS

One of the biggest success issues people encounter is staying on track and not rebounding back after they've achieved successful fat loss and reached their target goal. Section 3 of this book covers how to maintain healthy habits by focusing on emotional health. Here in the logistics section, I recommend a practical technique that you can use to assess yourself periodically, which I refer to as a checkpoint.

At the same time that you are setting your target fat loss goals, you should also set up "checkpoint goals" for yourself. First, you must make a commitment to yourself that you will actually carry out your checkpoint assessment. Just like you go to your doctor for regular physicals, you should monitor your checkpoint. Second, and the whole purpose of the checkpoint, is you must commit to not going past your checkpoint without taking action.

Here are some options for checkpoints:

1. The most accurate option is getting a body composition test that shows your visceral fat level and total body fat level. I like to use the visceral fat score because this elevates disease risk.

2. Waist circumference

3. Clothing size

4. Weight on a scale

🔹 EAT LESS

So, if you've determined that you have fat to burn, what's next? In order to get rid of fat effectively as you get older, you will need to reduce the number of calories you are consuming. Patients have come to me for years saying that they just don't understand why they are gaining weight when they have not changed the way they have eaten for years, but since they've reached a "certain age," they continue to slowly gain weight each year, always around the midsection. Some patients tell me that they had some initial success with changing their diet, even if they kept their calories about the same, and changed their macronutrient balance significantly, like going on a ketogenic diet. Those patients who switch to a balanced whole foods diet or anti-inflammatory diet from a standard American diet filled with processed foods will see some encouraging results initially. However, what is true in almost all of these cases is that the initial weight loss they experience is the result of water loss, and then their results, in terms of fat loss, often become disappointing. It's not until you cut calories that you will see significant changes in fat loss over time.

How to start eating less

Eating less seems like it should be straightforward, but I can offer some advice here that has worked well for many of my patients. First, download an app that allows you to track how many calories you're consuming daily. In order to do this accurately, you will need to measure your ingredients and portions. This process alone can be very revealing and powerful, seeing how many calories are in the foods you consume. Many people remark that they wouldn't have been eating as much if they knew how many calories they were consuming. This also helps you figure out where you may be able to cut calories that won't leave you feeling deprived. For example, reducing the amount of oil used in meal preparation is not something most people report missing. Also, when it comes to grains (more on grains in chapter 8), most people are exceeding a standard serving size, and those calories add up quickly.

Conquering overeating

In my book, *Unzip Your Genes*, I discussed behavioral techniques for addressing the gene variant for eating disinhibition. This common gene can increase your tendency to overeat and/or practice emotional or stress eating. Here are some of my favorite tips to conquer it:

* Recognize your triggers for emotional eating, and when you see one coming, have a substitute lined up. Find something other than food that elevates your mood—music, exercise, dancing, or talk to that friend who always makes you laugh!

* Don't buy those foods that are your saboteurs.

* Don't start eating the foods that you know you can't resist finishing. You really do need to practice avoidance.

* Measure or portion your foods, especially those that you really enjoy. You can't put a large piece of chocolate cake on your plate and say to yourself, "Oh, I'll just take a couple of bites."

* Continue to track your calories.

* Tell your friends, your partner, anyone who will listen!! Get it out in the open and you will feel so much relief. People can save you, especially in social settings. Ask them to "Keep me away from that buffet table" or "Don't offer me dessert."

Finding new foods that help control negative effects of bingeing

Many of us know the experience of going on a bender. I'm not talking about a drunken episode here—instead, a carb bender. The impact of stress that is not dealt with effectively, emotional upset, and disordered eating patterns can all lead to carb bingeing. Bigger-picture answers are working on stress and emotional health and regulating overall eating habits (as I am teaching you here). In the short term, when you have some options in the house for a controlled-effect binge, then you can shut down those cravings in a sitting.

The act of eating, chewing, and swallowing satisfies a lot of the craving. Finding foods that take a while to eat, don't set off the sugar receptors, but instead contain bitter bioactives, is the goal. One great and easy option is edamame, which may sound strange and not satisfying at first, but here's what it has going for it. First of all, buy a large bag of frozen, organic edamame that is not shelled. These don't go bad quickly, because they are in the freezer, and they take only a few minutes to heat up. When most people binge eat, they want to eat quickly. It takes a while to eat edamame, because you have to squeeze them out of the pods, and then your brain has time to catch up with the signals from your stomach that food has arrived. A large bowl of edamame is only about one hundred calories, very high in protein (about 12 grams), and is low carb. And, of course, soybeans bind the bitter receptors.

The initial discomfort of eating less

If you have excess fat stored and the goal is to burn that fat away, you have to prepare yourself for the fact that, initially, it will feel uncomfortable to eat less. As I now warn patients, when you reduce your calories there is a transitional period where you may feel the discomfort of eating less. As your body adjusts to the reduction in incoming fuel, those feelings (the ones that make you want to give up and scrap this new way of eating) will go away. You must be steady in your mindset and prepared to combat those physical and emotional feelings in order to power through the transition period. This transition period lasts about two to three weeks. Prepare your mind and willpower for this period of discomfort.

Feelings you may experience when you are reducing your calorie intake

If you have reduced your calories, you can feel some or all of these feelings and sensations during the transition period:

1. Irritable

2. Grumbling sounds in your stomach

3. Hunger pains

4. Empty sensation in your stomach

5. Intense cravings to eat…anything!

CHAPTER 7

The Bitter Prescription Dietary Essentials

*T*his chapter pulls together many of the topics I referenced in Section 1 that apply to dietary habits and provides some additional advice and considerations for adopting a healthier diet that better meets your digestive health and metabolic needs as you get older. The food lists are in the next chapter.

☞ GENERAL DIETARY GUIDELINES FOR THE BITTER PRESCRIPTION

Get more bitter bioactives in your diet

* Food quality is important: choose organic or heirloom produce that is produced locally and is as fresh as possible, whenever available.
* Grow some of your own food, at least fresh herbs.
* Diversity is key, eat a wide variety of foods.
* Add herbs and spices to your meals.

Be mindful of calories and glycemic impact

* Select foods rich in bitter bioactives, vitamins, and minerals, but not rich in calories.
* Choose lower glycemic impact foods, and eat foods low in added sugar—when you consume bitters, you tend to eat less sugar overall

Improve your digestion

    *   Drink concentrated bitters beverages before meals to stimulate adequate stomach acid production.

    *   Eat slowly.

    *   Don't drink too much along with meals because it may dilute gastric acid.

    *   Practice digestive rest.

Support your microbiota

    *   Eat foods that contain prebiotics and probiotics.

    *   Be mindful of fiber intake.

Food quality

Only a few generations back, our ancestors ate a diet that was rich in what I refer to as "living foods." The trendy concept of "farm to table" was just how people ate, and it wasn't restricted to those who could afford to eat in high-end restaurants. Unfortunately, now the conventional approach to food supply is largely dependent on international factory farming. This provides food that is less rich in bitters and bioactives. As you may remember from the first section, food scientists have long been developing cultivars of plants that are devoid of bitter compounds to meet the palatability of today's consumer, who has become more accustomed to the taste profile of the standard American diet, with the "side effect" being a deficit of healthful bitter bioactives.

Furthermore, we know that devoted organic farmers, who tend to the composition of their soil, produce plants with higher levels of health-promoting bioactives as well as higher amounts of minerals like magnesium. The health of the plant is also influenced by factors like music, different parts of the light spectrum, and even the emotional energy state of the gardener. I would strongly encourage you to eat more local, farm-fresh food if it is available to you. Consider joining a CSA, or start growing some of your own food, which can even be as simple as starting with growing herbs in a small garden bed or pots in your kitchen.

Diversity

One of my favorite quotes is by William Cowper: "Variety's the very spice of life, that gives it all its flavour." Although I imagine he wasn't thinking of the relationship between plants and microbial diversity, it can apply perfectly to this concept. Eating a broad range of plants—vegetables, fruits, legumes, herbs, and spices—is important for a healthy microbiome. Generally speaking, it's better to eat three cups of mixed green vegetables than four cups of all the same type. The unique compounds found in differing plants can promote growth of different types of commensal bacteria in the gut, which is what is referred to as microbial diversity. Many studies now suggest this is likely the most important hallmark of a healthy microbiota.

Bitter bioactives and calories

The next chapter lays out the foods that are concentrated in bitter bioactive compounds. The majority of these are plant foods, and many of these are also low calorie per serving (except for the categories that are marked with an asterisk). As I discussed in the previous chapter, if you need to shed excess fat stores, then it will be necessary to reduce your daily caloric intake, so you will need to be mindful of serving sizes and number of servings daily.

Low sugar and glycemic impact

To be as healthy as possible, you not only need to eat more dietary bitters, it's important to limit sugar intake. As I already explained, when you follow the Bitter Prescription and are consuming more bitters, your taste for sweet will change, and your strong cravings for sugar will dissipate. Furthermore, many people don't realize that the starches found in some vegetables, beans, and whole grains, if eaten in larger servings, can have a higher impact on blood sugar response, which is referred to as the glycemic impact.

Most of you are probably familiar with the distinction between good carbs and bad carbs, which is determined by a measurement called glycemic load (GL). When you eat food containing carbs, such as pasta, how much your blood sugar rises in response to a specific amount consumed results in a GL value. Lower glycemic load is desirable. Starches like instant rice, processed cereals, and flour products have the highest glycemic load, while starchy vegetables and some fruits (like bananas) have a moderate glycemic load, and non-starchy vegetables, beans, and most fruits have the lowest glycemic load. For this reason, I have separated the vegetables that are considered starchy on the vegetable food list in the next chapter. You should also take care with certain types of fruit, making sure you don't exceed the serving size and limit your servings per day.

Pay close attention to the starchy vegetables, beans, and grains categories, especially if you are trying to achieve fat loss, and make sure you follow these guidelines:

* Stick to the serving size.

* Separate these starches by meals to limit impact and provide satiety—in other words, don't eat rice and potatoes in the same meal.

* Rotate days for enhanced fat loss—that is, eat only one serving of starch daily.

Usually, our meals and snacks contain a combination of carbs, fat, and protein. The amounts of each can vary widely, which allows you to use the concept of food combinations to your advantage. The concept of food-combining alters the glycemic load of the meal. Consuming fats and proteins slows down the digestive process and reduces the glycemic load of the carbohydrates in the meal. Furthermore, fiber and water content also lower the glycemic load of the meal. Although an apple has a relatively low glycemic load, eating it with nuts (which contain healthy fats, some protein, and fiber) will further lower the effect on your blood sugar. When you're preparing meals and snacks, think about food combining, which is a very simple way of improving the glycemic impact.

Digestive function support
As I reviewed in the first part of the book, as we age, our digestive function declines. It is critical to support adequate digestion through a diet rich in bioactive bitters, but for many people, I recommend some extra measures to boost digestive capacity. There may be a benefit to including nutritional supplements to achieve optimal acid and enzyme levels (addressed in the digestive health chapter), but for many people, dietary sources alone may be adequate.

Beverages
When it comes to beverages, timing is important. Starting your day with bitter and drinking a bitter beverage just prior to your meal is a potent way to stimulate the bitter receptors and get your digestive system and metabolism ready for the incoming meal. Here are some examples:

* diluted apple cider vinegar (if more digestive distress)

* lemon water (not cold)

* tea, coffee (no cream or milk)

* bitter greens concentrate

Water

Staying hydrated throughout the day is very important. When you are incorporating bitter beverages into your diet, those will satisfy some of your daily water requirement. I recommend consuming the rest of your water between meals and during your digestive rest period. Drinking too much water with your meal could dilute your gastric juices and impair optimal digestion.

Eat slowly

Eating your meals too quickly is terrible for your digestion, allows you to gain weight more easily, and, research shows, can lead to a higher incidence of obesity and metabolic syndrome. When you slow down your eating, you become more in tune with the signals that you have eaten enough and will be less likely to overeat. When you eat too quickly, the satiety signals from your stomach that control appetite don't have enough time to communicate with your brain that you have eaten enough. It's also very important to spend enough time chewing your food thoroughly, because the process of chewing helps break down the food mechanically, gives the salivary enzymes adequate time to work on initial digestion, and the jaw reflex signals the rest of your digestive system for incoming food.

Eating style

In chapter 3, I reviewed the eating styles associated with obesity. I would encourage you to go back and take a look at those again and work on any that might be sabotaging your health. The main takeaways are:

* Respect the world that provides us sustenance.

* Express gratitude for nutritious, fresh food.

* Appreciate the surroundings in which you eat.

* Eat only when you are hungry.

* Take time to prepare nutritious meals.
* Enjoy meals in a relaxing atmosphere with people you love.
* Focus on your meal and no other tasks.

Order of eating

What you eat first in your meal may improve your digestive process. Ayurvedic diet planning often starts a meal with sipping warm water with lemon. The compounds found in lemon are strong bitters and can prepare the digestive process for improved assimilation of nutrients from your meal. What your taste buds sense first is important for improving digestion, specifically consuming bitters at the start of a meal. This may be lemon water or green tea, but it could be a small arugula salad dressed with fresh lemon or even bitter fruit, like grapefruit.

From the approach of improving blood sugar control, I have often recommended to my patients, if possible, depending on the makeup of their meals, to eat the concentrated protein and vegetables first before consuming the starch portion of the meal. For example, if you were having grilled salmon, asparagus, and roasted baby potatoes, start by eating the salmon and asparagus together, saving the potatoes for the end, or at least eat most of the salmon initially before beginning to work on the potatoes.

Digestive rest and eating window

Not eating for a minimum of fourteen hours, with the ideal being sixteen hours to improve insulin sensitivity, is what I refer to as digestive rest. This should ideally be practiced with an early cutoff time instead of a late start time, because nighttime eating has been shown to increase risk of obesity and diabetes. Depending on what time you get up in the morning, it could look like this:

* With a fourteen-hour fasting period: 8:00 a.m.–6:00 p.m.

* With a sixteen-hour fasting period: 9:00 a.m.–5:00 p.m.

When my patients are first starting out and they are eating all day long, right up until bedtime, I often suggest for them to ease into it by starting out with restricting eating within two hours before going to sleep. This alone can often relieve the nighttime indigestion that some people feel when they get into bed. As the body adapts to the metabolic and digestive rest, then the focus becomes increasing the fasting period to fourteen hours and possibly higher, depending on that person's overall health status. Also, don't graze during your eating window. It's important to space your meals due to the migratory motor complex (described in the chapter on digestion in section one).

*Warning: People with advanced diabetes and those on medications for diabetes, pregnant and breastfeeding moms, and people with eating disorders should not attempt intermittent fasting/digestive rest unless under close supervision of their physician.

Meal timing

I advise many of my patients to eat more of their calories earlier in the day, thereby front loading the day with dinner being a lighter meal. After a full night of sleep, stores of glutathione (our main antioxidant that protects our cells from DNA damage) are at their lowest, so flooding the system with a breakfast rich in glutathione and bioactives helps the body make more of its own glutathione. Fruits and vegetables are good sources. Again, evening eating raises the risk of obesity and diabetes.

Fiber

Fiber not only adds bulk to your diet, which is good for satiety, it also serves these roles:

* mechanical removal of damaged cells from the digestive tract

* a fermentable source for bacterial action, resulting in higher levels of short chain fatty acids (SCFAs), which are needed for a healthy microbiota

* increases stool bulk, dilutes carcinogens, and improves their transit time out of the body

* reduces cholesterol concentrations by inhibiting reabsorption of cholesterol

* binds estrogens and improves removal of estrogens through the stool

* lowers the glycemic impact of your meals

* enhances bowel motility

By following the Bitter Prescription, you should have no trouble meeting the dietary requirement of 25–35 grams of fiber daily.

Microbiome supportive foods

When you are choosing foods that contain bitter bioactives and eating using the diversity principle, you will already be supporting a healthy microbiome. But there are a group of plants that are particularly supportive because of their prebiotic content, providing more specialized support for the growth of healthy commensal bacteria. These are the microbiome superfoods:

* Asparagus
* Carrots
* Chickpeas
* Chocolate
* Dandelion greens
* Fermented foods: kimchi, miso
* Jerusalem artichoke
* Jicama
* Mushrooms
* Onions
* Radishes
* Tomatoes
* Turmeric

Interestingly, eating fresh, organic vegetables right out of the garden (what I refer to as living food) is also thought to provide some benefit. When I was a child, my brother and I had our own small vegetable garden. Of course, we ate the peas directly off the plant, but I remember pulling up carrots and only giving them a quick rinse outside before devouring them. We also routinely ate wild strawberries, blueberries, and blackberries (really any berry we knew was edible) right off the bushes and never got sick. Now, fast forward four decades later, and we have a lovely garden right outside our door filled with plants that my three kids will eat fresh out of the bed.

Cooking and food preparation techniques

Food preparation and cooking techniques can alter the bioactive content of plants. In general, cooking plants at high temperatures and for longer periods of time and microwaving depletes the bioactive content more than steaming and boiling. This does not mean you have to stop sautéing your vegetables. While it is not necessary to go on a completely raw foods diet, it is important to include some uncooked plants in your daily diet. This is easily accomplished by eating fresh fruit, some raw vegetables/salads, and adding fresh, uncooked herbs to your finished cooked dish.

CHAPTER 8

The Bitter Prescription Foods

This is the chapter with the food lists, which contain foods that are not only rich in bitter bioactives but are also supportive of overall digestive health and the microbiome. Because part of the Bitter Prescription includes eating less if you have excess fat to lose, I am indicating the foods for which the serving size should be limited, due to glycemic load and/or caloric density, with an asterisk (*). These categories are: starchy vegetables, fruit, legumes, nuts, seeds and oils, sweeteners, grains, concentrated protein. The foods lists are:

* Vegetables
* Fruit
* Fungus and Algae
* Legumes
* Nuts, Seeds, and Dietary Fats
* Herbs, Spices, and Condiments
* Beverages
* Concentrated Protein
* Grains

⟶ VEGETABLES

I am intentionally starting out with vegetables, as these should be an abundant and diverse part of your daily diet. Many people tend to get stuck in a rut of eating the same vegetables over and over. I would encourage you to start by going through the vegetable lists and checking off which ones you have eaten in the last thirty days. If you are like most people, you will be left with a hefty group of vegetables that you can add to your new grocery lists to get more plant variety in your diet. And remember, if you are a supertaster for bitter, as you add in some of the more mildly bitter-tasting foods, you will become more accustomed to the taste of bitter, and, over time, the very bitter-tasting foods won't taste so unpleasant to you. Make sure you are eating brassica or cruciferous vegetables daily as these are rich sources of glucosinolates.

I also advise people to rotate their vegetables on a regular basis. So if you bought kale this week, buy Swiss chard the next week. Also of note, younger sprouts concentrate the bioactives, so if you see these at the farmers market or grocery store, add them to your shopping bag. The vegetable list here is divided into non-starchy and starchy vegetables, because the starchy vegetables can spike your blood sugar levels if you eat too large a portion or too many servings daily. Ideally, only one serving of starchy vegetables daily is sufficient for most people. These can even be rotated every few days for people who are more aggressively working on reducing excess body fat. I don't place restrictions on the non-starchy vegetables and encourage the highest intake in this category.

Non-starchy vegetables
* Artichoke
* Arugula/rocket
* Asparagus (white is more bitter)

* Bamboo shoots
* Beet greens
* Bok choy
* Broccoli (or Calabrese, an Italian variety)
* Broccoli rabe
* Broccolini
* Brussels sprouts
* Cabbage (green, napa, red/purple, savoy)
* Cauliflower (green, orange, purple, and white varieties)
* Celeriac
* Collards
* Cucumber
* Daikon
* Dandelion greens
* Eggplant
* Escarole
* Fennel
* Fiddleheads
* Garlic
* Ginger
* Green beans (haricots verts, string, purple, wax, heirloom varieties)
* Jerusalem artichokes (sunchokes)
* Jicama
* Kale

* Kohlrabi
* Lettuce (bibb/Boston/butter, frisée, leaf—red and green, mâche, mesclun, romaine)
* Leek
* Microgreens
* Mustard greens
* Okra
* Onion (cipollini red, white, yellow)
* Peppers (banana, bell, jalapeno, poblano, shishito—too many to list here)
* Purslane
* Radicchio
* Radish
* Ramps
* Rhubarb
* Romanesco
* Scallion
* Shallot
* Snow peas
* Sorrel
* Spinach
* Sprouts
* Squash (delicata, spaghetti, yellow—the others are under starchy vegetables)
* Swiss chard
* Turnip greens
* Tomatillos

* Tomatoes
* Watercress
* Water chestnuts
* Zucchini

Starchy vegetables*

* Beet
* Carrot (orange, purple, red, yellow, white)
* Parsnip
* Potato (baby red/multicolor or Yukon gold)
* Pumpkin
* Sweet potato (orange and purple)
* Rutabaga
* Squash (acorn, butternut, hubbard)
* Turnip

*Limit serving size to one-half cup

⬤ FRUIT*

The fruit section is divided into berries and all other fruits. Berries are rich in a class of compounds called anthocyanins, and getting some berries in your diet daily is a great way to get a concentrated dose of antioxidants. My cousin and I look back at our childhood and think we would have been great foragers in another lifetime, because we spent our summers in Newfoundland eating wild berries of many varieties, most of which are not available commercially. We knew which ones were safe to eat and which ones were toxic. I recommend eating wild-sourced berries whenever you can, as they have higher levels of bitter bioactives. Again, you should rotate the types of berries and fruit you eat and take a seasonal approach as good quality fruit is not available year round. Frozen berries and fruit are still good options when fresh versions are not available.

Berries*

* Acai
* Cloudberry/bakeapple
* Bilberry
* Blueberry
* Blackberry
* Cape gooseberry
* Cherry
* Cranberry
* Currant (black, red, white)
* Goji
* Gooseberry
* Grape (black, green, red)
* Huckleberry
* Mulberry (black, lavender, purple, red, or white)
* Partridgeberry/lingonberry
* Persimmon
* Raspberry (black, golden, red, and white)
* Strawberry

*Limit serving size: about 1 cup contains 100 calories

Fruit*

* Apple (many varieties)—1 large
* Apricot—3
* Date—2
* Fig—2
* Grapefruit—1
* Grape—15
* Kiwi—2
* Kumquat—8
* Lemon
* Lime
* Mandarin (tangerines, satsumas)—2
* Mango—1/2 medium
* Melon (cantaloupe—1/2 medium, honeydew—1/4 small, watermelon—2 cups)
* Nectarine—2
* Orange (blood, cara cara, clementine, navel, tangelo, valencia)—1 large
* Papaya—1 1/2 cups
* Peach—2
* Pear—1
* Plum, Japanese (black, red and yellow)—2
* Plum, greengage—7
* Plum, Italian—3
* Pomegranate—1 1/2
* Pomelo—1/2

*Limit servings: serving sizes indicated above equate to about 100 calories

A word of caution about grapefruit

The levels of certain medications can be affected by consuming grapefruit, resulting in higher blood levels of your medication and the potential of adverse effects. In some cases, it can decrease the blood level, making the medication less effective. You should check with the pharmacist about your specific medicines and whether it is ok to incorporate grapefruit regularly into your diet.

Notes

* In general, try to avoid overripe fruit. The more immature a fruit is, the higher the concentration of bitter compounds.

* Always eat the peel if edible, because it typically contains high levels of bioactives.

* Eat the pith on citrus as it is a rich source of bitters.

* Add grated citrus peel to recipes.

➡ FUNGUS AND ALGAE*

Here's a pretty unique part of the Bitter Prescription. I recommend eating fungus and algae daily. This might sound strange at first, and you might think it's even a bit wacky, but these specific foods that I am recommending are rich sources of bioactive compounds. The types of fungus I am referring to are mushrooms and certain types of moldy cheeses that are good for your gut flora. Obviously, if you have a dairy allergy or are lactose intolerant, dairy sensitive, or vegan, then I would not say you must start eating cheese, but, instead, you should focus on the mushrooms. Also, you do not need to eat these moldy cheeses daily, as they are dense in calories. Instead, eat them up to a few times per week. There are many types of mushrooms, and they are known to have great benefits for the immune system. Again, I recommend diversity. Some mushroom varieties are very expensive and not widely available, but even small amounts provide benefits. If you are making a mushroom dish, you can use inexpensive creminis as the base and add in smaller amounts of shiitakes or chanterelles. Grocery stores often stock packaged fresh multi-mushroom mixes, and those are a good option to gain more diversity. Some mushroom varieties can be seasonal, so keep an eye out for new ones at your local grocer.

As for the algae advice, here, I am referring to sea vegetables, which are not only a great source of bioactives but also rich in trace minerals. These can be added to salad, and dried powdered versions of arame and dulse (widely available in a seasoning shaker) can be added to soups and stews.

Mushrooms and truffles

* Black trumpet/black chanterelle
* Beech/honshimeiji
* Bluefoot
* Button
* Chanterelle
* Chicken of the woods
* Cremini
* Enoki
* Hedgehog
* Lion's mane
* Oyster
* Maitake/hen of the woods
* Morels

* Porcini
* Portobello
* Shiitake
* Trumpet Royale/king trumpet/king oyster
* Truffle (black and white varieties)
* Wood ear

Moldy cheese*

Only certain types of cheese that are intentionally meant to contain mold are what I am referring to here. Cheeses that have gone bad in your fridge like cottage cheese, cream cheese, ricotta, or grated cheese should be thrown away. If you are a cheese aficionado, you will appreciate the taste of a great blue cheese that makes your tongue feel almost numb. Many cheeses are also started with a yeast culture. The most common moldy cheeses are:

* English Stilton
* French Roquefort
* Italian Gorgonzola
* French Époisses

*Limit serving size: 1 oz. contains about 100 calories

Sea vegetables

Often thought of as "plants of the sea," the correct classification for sea vegetables is algae. Japan has a very rich history of eating sea vegetables, and these are a staple of the traditional Japanese diet. They are very rich in trace minerals, a well-known source of iodine, and also contain bitter bioactives. The most common sea vegetable eaten in America is nori, which is the greenish-black wrapper used to make sushi rolls.

* Arame
* Dulse
* Hijiki
* Kelp
* Kombu
* Nori

⬤ LEGUMES*

Legumes are another category that, while they contain powerful bitter bioactives, also need to be eaten in moderation. Because they contain complex carbohydrates, the calories can add up quickly, and when eaten in too large a serving size, or too many servings, they can impact blood sugar control.

Legumes*

* Adzuki
* Black
* Black-eyed pea
* Cannellini (white Italian kidney bean)
* Cranberry/borlotti beans
* Fava
* Flageolet
* Garbanzo/chickpea
* Great northern bean
* Green pea
* Hummus—1/4 cup
* Kidney

* Lentil (black/beluga, brown, green/French, red, yellow)
* Lima (butter, baby lima)
* Mung
* Navy
* Pinto
* Soybean/edamame
* Yellow split pea

*Limit serving size: 1/2 cup cooked legumes (100 cal), 3/4 cup soup (100 cal), unless indicated

➡ Nuts, Seeds, and Dietary Fats*

While nuts and seeds have a very low glycemic impact, because of their high fat content, calories add up quickly, so serving size on these really matters. Nuts and seeds are an amazing source of phytochemicals. They are also rich in healthy fats, fiber, and minerals. For example, Brazil nuts contain a specific form of the trace mineral selenium called selenomethionine, which is important for a balanced immune system. Concentrated oils and fats contain bioactives and are also part of a healthy diet but must be used in moderation due to their high caloric density.

Nuts*

* Almond
* Brazil nut
* Cashew
* Chestnut
* Coconut (technically a fruit, but here due to its fat content)

* Hazelnut
* Macadamia
* Marcona almond
* Nut butter
* Peanut (technically a legume, but due to its fat content included here)
* Pecan
* Pistachio
* Walnut

Seeds*

* Chia
* Flax
* Hemp/hemp heart
* Pine nut
* Poppy
* Pumpkin
* Sesame
* Sunflower

*Limit serving size to equate to about 100 calories, check nutrition label—varies widely

Concentrated oils and fats*

* Avocado (1/8)
* Avocado oil
* Flaxseed oil (don't use for cooking)

* Olives (8–10 medium)—many varieties such as Kalamata, Ligurian, Manzanilla, Niçoise, Picholine
* Extra virgin olive oil, herb-infused olive oil
* Sesame oil/hot pepper sesame oil
* Walnut oil (don't use for cooking)

*Limit serving size: one serving is 1 teaspoon of oil (equates to about 40 calories), others indicated above

⬤ HERBS, SPICES, AND CONDIMENTS

Herbs and spices hold a dear place in my heart, and I cannot imagine what my diet would be like without these potent plants. Earlier in my career, I was appointed as the medical editor for the *Journal of Herbs, Spices and Medicinal Plants,* and I was so lucky to get a firsthand look at the amazing research taking place internationally. Herbs and spices can be used lavishly without regard for calories, but it doesn't take much to have an effect on the flavor of food, as well as our metabolism. Condiments are another way to get more diversity of phytochemicals and flavor in the diet.

Herbs and Spices

* Allspice
* Anise
* Basil
* Bay leaf
* Caraway
* Cardamom
* Celery seed

* Chervil
* Chile (many types)
* Chive
* Chocolate
* Cilantro
* Cinnamon
* Cloves
* Coriander
* Cumin
* Dill
* Fennel seed
* Fenugreek
* Galangal
* Garlic
* Ginger
* Lavender
* Lemongrass
* Marjoram
* Mint
* Mustard
* Nigella
* Nutmeg
* Oregano
* Paprika
* Parsley
* Peppercorn (black, green, red, white)

* Rosemary
* Saffron
* Sage
* Savory
* Star anise
* Sumac
* Tarragon
* Thyme
* Turmeric
* Vanilla

Condiments

* Aioli* (watch fat content/calories)
* Capers
* Chutneys and relishes* (watch sugar content)
* Coarse ground Dijon mustard
* Cornichons/gherkins
* Giardiniera—or Italian pickled vegetables
* Harissa
* Hoisin
* Horseradish
* Hot sauce
* Miso
* Pesto
* Pickled vegetables
* Salsa
* Sriracha

* Tahini
* Tamari/soy sauce
* Vinegars
* Wasabi
* Worcestershire

Sweeteners*

* Agave*
* Blackstrap molasses*
* Date syrup*
* Honey*
* Monk fruit
* Stevia

*Limit serving size to 1 tsp.

There is more to these sweeteners than just sugar. There are other beneficial compounds that can actually have a positive impact on human health. For example, blackstrap molasses (BSM) is rich in polyphenols, which have powerful effects on our DNA. It can increase gene expression for several liver and fat cell biomarkers of energy metabolism, thereby impacting how we use calories. But even more interesting is that BSM reduces the number of calories we absorb, serving double duty. An animal study looked at two groups, both fed the same high fat diet, but one supplemented with molasses. At the end of twelve weeks, the molasses group had a lower body weight, decreased fat mass, and lower levels of a hormone called leptin that impacts fat metabolism. This is a simple study that discounts the calorie theory and sugar-free diets, while lending support to a return to sensible, traditional eating. Molasses contains four grams of sugar per teaspoon, the same amount as table sugar, but it has a lower glycemic index, and it contains all the goodness from the whole sugar cane that was stripped away from the table sugar. This is what makes it one of the better sweeteners.

For obvious reasons, it is important to not go overboard on sugar consumption, but, occasionally, when there is a desire to add a sweetener to something you are preparing, it's nice to know what the best options are. When it comes to honey, there are many types of honey available. Some, like Jamun, have a lower glycemic impact than others. Also to consider is that certain types of honey, such as Greek honey, are richer in bioactive compounds.

Living herbs

If you live in a climate where you can grow herbs outside, year round, I am jealous! For those of us who have a cold winter, in order to have access to living herbs, we need to grow them inside. The good news is that growing herbs is easy, it takes up little space, as you can grow a bunch in the same pot, and they are not time consuming to care for. You can grow them from seeds or just purchase organic potted herbs. Your herb garden becomes your daily punch of living food.

These herbs are easy to grow indoor herbs:

* Basil

* Chives

* Mint

* Oregano

* Parsley

* Rosemary

* Sage

* Thyme

● BEVERAGES

Your choice in beverages can also have an impact on the bitter taste system. Activating the bitter receptors prior to eating is a great way to enhance the digestive process, getting the body ready for incoming food.

Tea

In general, Japanese green tea contains the most bitter bioactive compounds. The longer you steep your tea, the more of these phytochemicals are extracted from the leaves. The practice of drinking the first extraction after a few minutes and then re-steeping can pull out more of these compounds. Another option is to just let your tea steep longer—at least five minutes. I tend to just leave my tea bag in my large cup and sip on it throughout the morning. Research has shown that drinking green tea can improve your metabolism and may help with weight loss.

Matcha green tea

Matcha is a sensory and, for some, even a spiritual experience, as it may be drunk near meditation. The complexity of this ancient beverage is part of what makes this tea so wonderful. Matcha has gained popularity in the United States as a healthy source of concentrated antioxidants, resulting in the trendy matcha latte prepared with cream and sugar. However, the traditional way to consume matcha is preferable, mixed simply with water and sipped quickly from a small bowl, as some of the powder will come out of the solution. Matcha tastes bitter and malty with an undertone of seaweed flavor. (See the recipes chapter for instructions on how to prepare matcha.)

Black tea

Black tea also contains bitter compounds. You should avoid adding milk to your tea, though, because it binds up those health-promoting flavonols. There was even a study that showed that the weight loss effects were blunted when milk was added to tea. Like with green tea, you can also re-steep it to pull out more of the bioactive compounds, or simply leave it steeping longer. Earl Gray tea is a favorite of mine, and its distinctive flavor comes from the addition of bergamot oil, which comes from the peel of the bitter Italian citrus fruit, touted for heart heath. Pu-erh and oolong tea also have similar health promoting properties.

Coffee

Recent research has shown, if you are less sensitive to bitterness, you're more likely to drink coffee, while if you're more sensitive to the taste of bitter compounds, then you are more likely to drink tea. Similar to tea, it's better to take your coffee black, because the addition of milk or cream binds up those beneficial bitter compounds, mainly the polyphenols. I recommend drinking sustainable and organically grown coffee, ideally espresso, which is high in bitter compounds, but lower in caffeine than drip-brewed coffee. If you're drinking coffee (or tea) when you first get up in the morning and practicing digestive rest, then this is another reason not to put cream in your coffee, because it would break the extended overnight fast.

Herbal teas (caffeine-free)

Herbal teas are made up of medicinal plants, and they all have bitter compounds in them, some more than others. Herbal teas for digestive health tend to have herbs with more of an affinity for improving digestive function, especially easing gas and bloating. This action is referred to as carminative. Bitter carminative herbs are also available in capsule form. Here are some of my favorite digestive herbal teas (all of which are commercially available as herbal blends as well):

* Angelica
* Chamomile
* Chai (this is my go-to natural caffeine-free tea and contains a base of cinnamon, cardamom, cloves)
* Chicory
* Dandelion
* Fennel
* Gentian
* Ginger
* Lemon balm
* Peppermint

A word about caffeine

Some people have medical conditions, like heart problems, for which caffeine intake is to be avoided. Although caffeine itself does taste bitter, there are so many other bitter compounds found in decaffeinated tea and coffee, herbal teas, and, of course, all throughout the plant kingdom, that there is no concern for health detriment by avoiding caffeine. Furthermore, for many people who are slow metabolic processors of caffeine (which can be determined through genetic testing), I recommend drinking no more than one cup per day of coffee. The average cup of coffee contains 100 mg of caffeine. If you are a tea drinker, caffeine content is much lower, on the order of 25–40 mg per cup, so you can handle a couple of cups.

Bitter tonics

For more intensive digestive support, I may recommend adding a bitter tonic just before the meal to enhance the digestive process.

* Apple cider vinegar (ACV) tonic—1–3 teaspoons ACV (mix 1:1 with water)
* Lemon water—1/2 lemon juiced in a few ounces of warm water
* Tonic water (sugar free) which contains the bitter compound quinine—2–3 ounces
* Herbal bitters—1/4 teaspoon straight or mixed in few ounces of warm water (available commercially)

Water

In general, I recommend following the traditional naturopathic and Ayurvedic practices of limiting the amount of water you consume along with your meals, as it may make the digestive process in the stomach less effective. Instead, make sure you drink most of your daily water between meals.

Alcoholic beverages

Alcohol consumption and health outcomes is a controversial topic, because there are conflicting studies on alcohol intake and disease risk. There are studies that show reduced risk of heart disease with moderate alcohol consumption (defined as one drink per day for women, two drinks for men). In my practice, I do not recommend daily drinking for generally healthy people. Instead, and only if desired, occasional moderate alcohol consumption, for those who have no contraindications, may confer some health benefits.

There are quite a few conditions for which alcohol intake is ill advised (this is not a complete list), including people on certain medications, those with liver disease, some types of heart disease, diabetes, personal (or family) history of certain cancers and mood disorders, pregnancy, and nursing mothers. Across the board, heavy drinkers (defined as eight or more drinks per week for women) have higher risks of mortality and many diseases, including high blood pressure, heart failure, stroke and liver disease. Of course, if you have dealt with alcohol abuse or avoid alcohol because of family history of alcohol abuse, I would not encourage you to start drinking. As with caffeine, there are many other sources of bitter bioactives throughout the plant kingdom that can provide benefit without needing to include alcohol as part of your lifestyle.

Apéritifs, bitters, and spirits

Alcoholic bitters were very popular in the 1800s and were often served as an apéritif, added to pre-dinner cocktails, or as a digestif, served after dinner to improve digestion. These cocktail ingredients are essentially neutral spirits that have been infused with aromatics, such as spices, tree bark, roots, seeds, and fruits. The next time you go out for drinks with friends, scan the cocktail menu to look for bitter drinks like the classic Negroni. Some common examples of bitter spirits include:

* Angostura
* Aperol
* Campari
* Herbal-infused spirits like craft gin

Wine

The main bioactive class of compounds found in red wine are called polyphenols and are made up of flavonols, anthocyanins, and the more widely recognized bioactive resveratrol, which is known for its antioxidant and anti-aging effects. These compounds contribute to the bitter tones and astringency of wine. Interestingly, the bitterness of phenolic compounds in grape skin and seeds (not much is found in the juice) is enhanced by alcohol but reduced by sugar. This is why wine and grape juice taste drastically different on the bitter scale. Research has shown that supertasters for bitter consume less red wine. Another note on wine is that, as wine ages, the main bitter bioactives, resveratrol, flavonols and anthocyanins tend to decrease, so heavily aged wines may not possess the same health value. There are so many options for wines available in the marketplace, and the complexity of wine is so immense. Generally speaking, when selecting wine, try to choose those produced from traditional approach—old-fashioned wineries who are not employing chemists to engineer the wines to save aging time, which reduces the level of resveratrol.

Beer

Earlier in this book, I mentioned hops, an ingredient in beer, as having a strong effect on the bitter taste receptors. In fact, bitterness in beer is such an important, and desirable, characteristic that there is a bitter scale that was devised early in the twentieth century, specifically for the beer industry, called the IBU, for International Bitterness Unit. It is a chemical measurement of the number of bitter compounds, including the aforementioned iso-alpha acids and polyphenols, that contribute to the bitter taste of beer. The bitters in beer come mainly from hops and malt. I imagine you're already wondering, "Which ones are the most bitter?" Somewhat similar to wine, beer is a complex beverage, and a higher bitter scale does not necessarily mean that the beer *tastes* more bitter than one with a lower rating. But luckily, that scale does tell us the level of bitter compounds, which, as you know by now, is more important for the potential health benefits than how bitter it tastes. Generally speaking, beer types with the highest IBU tend to be Imperial IPA, Imperial Stout, followed by American IPA, English IPA, and American Stout.

➡ CONCENTRATED PROTEIN*

Whether you eat a completely plant-based diet or you include dairy, eggs, seafood, and/or meats in your diet, the important thing is to make sure you are getting enough protein, but not too much. Your needs will vary according to your activity level, gender, current weight, and age (as you get older you need more protein because not as much is absorbed). Most people need a minimum of three servings per day.

Soy-derived protein is the highest in bioactive compounds. Genistein and daidzein are the main bioactive compounds that exert bitterness in soy. The process of making soy products like soy milk, tofu, and miso, whereby the first step is soaking the soybeans, enhances the bitter compounds. Fortunately, soy-based foods don't impart an extremely bitter taste like other plants and are a very nice addition to the diet. Make sure when you are choosing soy products to select the more traditionally consumed ones like tofu (instead of highly processed products with added soy protein) and to always buy organically grown. Many traditionally produced, old-world-style cheeses and yogurts can contain some bitter bioactives and are a part of the Mediterranean diet. Fish and meats are not good sources of bitters.

Protein*

* Beef (grass fed)—3–4 oz.
* Cheese—feta and other sheep cheeses like Manchego, goat, parmesan—1–2 oz.
* Egg—2 large
* Fish and shellfish—3–6 oz.
* Poultry—3–4 oz.
* Tofu—1 cup
* Tempeh—1/2 cup
* Yogurt (plain, whole milk traditionally prepared)—6 oz.

*Limit serving size: one serving is about 150 calories, indicated above, varies according to cut/fat content

⬤ GRAINS*

* Amaranth (GF)
* Barley
* Black rice (GF)
* Buckwheat (GF)
* Bulgur
* Bread—Ezekiel/Sprouted, Rye, Sourdough
* Millet (GF)
* Oats (GF)
* Pasta—black bean, chickpea, red lentil, soybean blends preferable
* Quinoa (GF)
* Teff (GF)
* Rice—basmati, brown, jasmine (GF)
* Red rice (GF)
* Wild rice (GF)
* GF—gluten free

*Limit serving size: one-half cup cooked whole grains or one slice of bread is about 100 calories.

A word (actually many words) on whole grains

When I was in medical school, we studied and practiced nutritional medicine in our student clinic. Dietary and lifestyle changes were at the core of what we taught our patients. I don't ever remember recommending a grain-free diet, except in cases where we prescribed a ketogenic diet as a medical diet for managing epilepsy (reports of the effectiveness of ketogenic diets for epilepsy go as far back as the 1920s). Instead, we instructed patients on how to implement a whole foods diet, with plenty of colorful vegetables, beans and lentils, nuts and seeds, healthy fats and oils, lean protein (vegetarian, fish and/or meats)...and *whole grains!* And you know what? Our patients felt better. They had more energy. They had reduced sugar cravings. They lost weight, and they had more regular bowel movements.

Fast forward about twenty years, and everywhere you turn, the dietary advice from all the latest gurus is mostly grain-free...forever! "Grains are toxic," we are told. But are there any life-long studies on people who eat grain-free diets to know what could happen to our overall health?

Furthermore, I am at the point now where I have observed enough patients on grain-free diets in my clinic that I am becoming convinced that this type of diet is not sustainable for most people. The trend I see is that people tend to cycle on and off of these diets and end up weighing more than they did when they started, and they often find that they no longer lose any weight or feel a difference when they go back to a strict grain-free diet. Bottom line is that grain-free diets might help you lose weight initially, but there is no evidence that they are good for your health long-term; actually, based on newer evidence, quite the contrary.

Eating whole grains reduces the risk of death from *all* causes

Two major meta-analysis prospective studies published in 2016 in very respectable medical journals, *Circulation* and *The BMJ*, demonstrated very clearly that consumption of whole grains reduces the risk of coronary artery disease, cardiovascular disease, total cancer, and the risk of dying from *all* causes. In one of the papers, the researchers pooled data from fourteen eligible studies, including almost eight hundred thousand people with nearly one hundred thousand deaths, while the second paper examined the results from forty-five cohort studies (meaning massive amounts of data was analyzed). In both studies, the conclusion was a robust positive impact on health from eating whole grains.

The most widely studied diet for cardiovascular health, diabetes, and reduction of all-cause mortality is the Mediterranean diet. And what does it consist of? Healthy fats from olive oil, nuts and seeds, poultry, eggs, seafood, lots of colorful fruits and vegetables, legumes, and *whole grains*. The Mediterranean diet has been shown to improve the pattern of DNA expression to influence genes associated with inflammation and fat metabolism.

What are you missing out on when you skip whole grains?
Whole grains contain a multitude of naturally occurring, health-promoting compounds. Many people recognize whole grains to be a rich source of dietary fiber. Whole grains are also a good source of magnesium, which can improve insulin sensitivity and reduce blood pressure. Other minerals in whole grains include iron, zinc, selenium, and copper. And, of course (you may have guessed it already), there are bioactive compounds like carotenoids and polyphenols in whole grains, which can impact gene expression and bind bitter receptors.

Why are people who eat whole grains less likely to die?
The health benefits of whole grains can be attributed to a number of factors. Certainly, the types of bioactive compounds and fiber in whole grains have the effects I have already outlined. A second finding is that people who eat whole grains have lower levels of inflammatory markers, like CRP, which is the opposite of what you are hearing out there about whole grains. In fact, the results from the Iowa Women's Health Study showed that women who eat whole grains are less likely to die from inflammatory diseases beyond cardiovascular disease and cancer, such as infectious diseases, respiratory diseases, and diseases of the digestive system.

Which unique bioactive compounds are found in whole grains?

What defines a whole grain is the presence of the germ, endosperm, and bran portions, as opposed to refined grains which only contain the endosperm. The bioactive compounds are found primarily in the bran/germ portion, which helps to explain why only whole grains can have such a tremendous impact on our healthspan. The main bioactives in whole grains are phenolic compounds, phytosterols, tocols, dietary fibers (mainly beta-glucan), lignans, alkylresorcinols, phytic acid, γ-oryzanols, avenanthramides, cinnamic acid, ferulic acid, inositols, and betaine. Some of these are found in other plants, but many are uniquely found only in whole grains in high levels, and some only in certain grains. For example, avenanthramides are found specifically in oats and have anti-inflammatory, anti-atherogenic, and antioxidant properties. Plant sterols are found in much higher levels in whole grains and can reduce cholesterol. Multiple studies have also shown plant sterols to help with colon cancer prevention. Gamma-oryzanol found in whole grain rice is a powerful antioxidant and is an effective treatment for hyperlipidemia, menopausal symptoms, and can help increase muscle mass.

Summary on eating whole grains

Research is continuing to show us the power of food as medicine. Skipping a major source of phytochemicals by choosing to eat grain-free for the rest of your life may not be a wise decision. Of course, in this era of factory farming with the widespread use of pesticides and other chemicals used in food production, we must be aware that some of the ill effects of dietary factors on our health may be attributed to food that is essentially 'unnatural'. As with any other foods, whenever possible, it's important to choose foods that are grown organically, the way nature intended.

CHAPTER 9

Menu Planning

$\mathcal{I}$ previously discussed the concept of digestive rest, wherein you don't eat for fourteen hours per day (most of this time is when you are sleeping anyway). The benefits of taking a break before bed can do wonders for your digestive and metabolic health. If you are planning to incorporate digestive rest into most of your days, then I would encourage you to set up your daily eating times to allow for plenty of rest prior to bedtime. For example, I get up between 5:30–6:00 a.m., typically start eating food around 8:30 a.m., and stop eating somewhere between 4:30–6:30 p.m. This gives me fourteen to sixteen hours of digestive rest. Some days, this type of schedule may not work for you, and it's fine if you don't get digestive rest every single day.

Here, I am sharing some examples of daily menu plans. Depending on how much you currently weigh, your age, how much you exercise, whether you are trying to lose weight, your health status, and so on, your caloric requirements will vary quite a bit. For best results, incorporating body composition testing (as I discussed in chapter 6 on fat loss) is one of the best ways to help determine exactly how much you need to eat daily and then plan your serving sizes accordingly. Using an app that tracks macronutrients and calories is really helpful in the early stages as you are making these dietary changes.

The beauty of the Bitter Prescription is that you can draw inspiration from many different cultures and cuisines. Because one of the keys to this plan is following the principle of diversity, the meals you end up eating daily can be very different from someone else who is also following the Bitter Prescription. In the next chapter, I offer some of my favorite recipes to give you ideas of meals you can plan that include ingredients with bitter bioactives. You can easily adapt many of your favorite recipes and meals to increase the amount and types of bitters you consume daily.

Meals don't need to be complex or have you spending a ton of time in the kitchen. When I am preparing recipes, I try to make them in larger quantities so I can use them for the meal at hand, but then it can also become lunch or part of other meals during the week.

SAMPLE MENU 1

- Morning beverage
    - * Black coffee
- Breakfast
    - * Peppermint tea
    - * Chia spice pudding with berries
- Morning snack
    - * Granny Smith apple and almonds
- Lunch
    - * Lemongrass and bergamot tea
    - * Mediterranean salad with grilled chicken
- Dinner
    - * Bitter tonic
    - * Arame-avocado spinach salad
    - * Roasted salmon and root vegetables

- Evening
  - * Ginger tea

SAMPLE MENU 2

- Morning beverage
  - * Earl Grey tea
- Breakfast
  - * Lemon water tonic
  - * Oatmeal with walnuts and fresh blackberries
- Snack
  - * Green smoothie with collagen
- Lunch
  - * Green tea
  - * Minestrone soup
- Dinner
  - * Watercress salad
  - * Herb roasted chicken, Provençal mushrooms, and mashed cauliflower
- Evening beverage
  - * Chamomile tea

SAMPLE MENU 3

- Breakfast
  - * Black coffee

- * Grapefruit and berries
- * Veggie omelet
- * Whole grain toast
- Lunch
  - * Green tea
  - * Greek cod
  - * Arugula salad with lemon
- Snack
  - * Sliced pear and blue cheese
- Dinner
  - * Chai tea
  - * Spicy red lentil soup
- Evening beverage
  - * Passionflower tea

CHAPTER 10

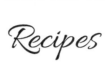
Recipes

$\mathcal{T}$his is, by far, not an attempt at delivering a mini cook-book. Instead, I wanted to share with you some of my favorite recipes and easy ways to get more bitter bioactives into your diet. I have always had a love of cooking. I enjoy preparing meals for my family (sometimes elaborate, and often not), entertaining friends with delicious and nutritious food, and I love the holidays, so I tend to go all out. I am often experimenting with new recipes. By reviewing these recipes, you will start to see familiar ingredients and themes. Then, as you skim through recipes online, look at your cookbooks, and family recipes, and watch cooking programs, you will be better equipped to pick the recipes that support the Bitter Prescription. With that said, let me start with some of my tips for stocking your pantry, followed by recipes to get you thinking about delicious ways to incorporate bitters in your diet.

➡ PANTRY BASICS

Time to stock your pantry. Get acquainted with your local grocer's bulk section. You can also order from online retailers. A good idea is to invest in a variety of sizes of mason jars, an inexpensive and toxin-free storage solution. Large mason jars are great to store beans, grains, nuts, and seeds. You can even use these jars as indoor containers to grow herbs.

Fortified salt
Many people are using specialty salts like sea salt and Himalayan salt for their touted health benefits, which is great, but

these types of salt are not iodized, and iodine is an essential nutrient that we can't make in our bodies, making us dependent on dietary sources. Iodine is necessary for healthy thyroid function, and I routinely find deficient blood levels in many of my patients. Here's a way of getting around that problem, without having to use standard iodized salt.

* 8 oz. Celtic or Himalayan salt
* 1 oz. kelp powder

• Blend with small whisk or stir well with a spoon until completely incorporated and use it the same way you would use standard salt.

Herb and spice blends

For ease, you can purchase pre-made spice blends, or you can mix your own. A rule of thumb is to make sure there are five or more ingredients in your spice blend to kick up your diversity.

Here are some common blends you can store in your pantry:

* Curry (turmeric, chili powder, coriander, cumin, ginger, and pepper)
* Dukkah (walnuts, hazelnuts, sesame seeds, coriander, cumin, salt, and pepper)
* Five spice powder (cinnamon, fennel, cloves, star anise, and pepper)
* Herbes de Provence (basil, fennel, lavender, marjoram, parsley, rosemary, savory, tarragon, and thyme)
* Italian seasoning (basil, marjoram, oregano, rosemary, and thyme)

* Old Bay Seasoning (celery salt, black pepper, crushed red pepper flakes, and paprika)

* Za'atar (oregano, thyme, marjoram, sesame seeds, and sumac)

Teas
Visit your local natural foods store and stock up on green tea, black tea, and herbal teas so you have plenty of options to add more diversity to your daily diet.

Preparing matcha green tea
You need a small ceramic bowl and a whisk. Add 1/4 tsp. of organic matcha powder with 10 oz. of hot water. Whisk vigorously for two minutes. Swirl and sip as you drink, because the matcha powder tends to settle to the bottom of the cup if it sits too long.

➥ SALADS AND DRESSINGS

Simple oil and vinegar dressing
I dress many of my single-serving green salads directly with only a very good extra virgin olive oil (one teaspoon) and balsamic vinegar (scant teaspoon) or juice from half a lemon, then sprinkling with a little salt. If it's just for me, I'm not mixing up a jar of dressing. However, if I'm serving a green salad for my family or friends, then I tend to use the following recipe, changing the herbs and acid depending on what I'm serving with it.

Herb salad dressing

* 2/3 cup fresh mixed herbs, chopped (basil, mint, thyme, parsley, thyme, chives, rosemary)

* one clove fresh garlic, crushed

* zest of one lemon
* 1/3 cup fresh lemon juice
* 2/3 cup olive oil
* 1/2 tsp. salt and freshly ground pepper

• Add lemon juice and olive oil, lemon zest, garlic, salt, and pepper to a small jar, cover, and shake. Uncover, add in the fresh herbs, and place cover back on and shake again.

Arame-avocado green salad

This is an easy, and delicious, way to get a dose of sea vegetables in your diet. Arame is a pretty mild-tasting seaweed that adds great texture to this salad.

* 1/8 cup dry arame, soaked in 1 cup of water for about fifteen min.
* 5 cups of spinach (or mesclun)
* one avocado, chopped into thin slices
* 1/4 red or orange bell pepper, thinly sliced
* 1/3 cup toasted almonds, chopped (roast dry on a cookie sheet at 350°F for about 5 min)
* 4 Tb. toasted sesame oil
* 3 Tb. brown rice vinegar
* 1 1/2 Tb. honey
* 1 Tb. course ground mustard
* 1 Tb. poppy seeds
* 1/2 tsp. salt

• Whisk together oil, vinegar, honey, mustard, poppy seeds, and salt in the bottom of a large bowl. Add the almonds and stir around. Then, add the spinach or salad greens, avocado, pepper, and drained arame and toss to coat with the dressing.

Arugula, lemon, and shaved parmesan

A very simple salad, this one works well as a meal appetizer and is great way to stimulate the bitter taste receptors prior to your entree.

* 2 cups arugula
* 1/2 lemon juiced, plus lemon zest (if desired)
* 1 scant tsp. olive oil
* 1/2 oz. shaved parmesan
* 1/8 tsp. salt

• Toss arugula in a bowl with lemon juice, olive oil, and salt. Top with shaved parmesan.

Asparagus and pea salad

This is one of my favorite salads to make when asparagus first comes out in the spring.

* 1 1/4 lb. thin asparagus, one-inch pieces
* one medium cucumber (sliced into quarters)
* 1/2 leek, halved and thinly sliced
* 1 cup green peas, fresh or thawed
* one avocado, cut into small chunks
* 1/4 cup fresh parsley, chopped
* 1 Tb. olive oil
* zest of one lemon
* 1 Tb. lemon juice
* one large clove garlic, crushed
* 1/2 tsp. salt and pepper

1. Blanche asparagus for three minutes and place in an ice bath.

2. Mix olive oil, lemon juice, garlic, and salt and pepper in the bottom of a large bowl that you will keep the salad in.

3. Add all the vegetables, cucumber, leek, peas, asparagus, avocado, and parsley to the bowl and toss to combine with the dressing on the bottom of the bowl.

Easy chickpea salad

This salad can often be found in my fridge. It makes a good addition for a packed lunch, and it serves as a satisfying snack. My kids will even eat a little bowl of this as an afternoon snack.

* two 15oz. cans of chickpeas/garbanzo beans
* lime zest
* juice of 1/2 lime
* 1 tsp. olive oil
* 1/4 tsp. salt
* 1/4 cup fresh parsley (optional)

• Drain and rinse chickpeas and place in a serving bowl. Add lime zest, lime juice, olive oil, salt pepper, and parsley and toss well.

Mediterranean salad

This is one of my go-to lunch salads. The measurements are for a single big salad, and you can assemble it directly on the plate.

* 2–3 cups lettuce/arugula base/fresh herbs
* 6 quarters marinated artichokes

* 1/2 cup fresh mixed vegetables (tomatoes, cucumber, peppers etc.)
* 1/4 cup chickpeas
* 1/8 cup feta
* 1/2 lemon juiced over salad, or 1 tsp. vinegar
* 1 tsp. extra virgin olive oil

You can serve this with 2–3 oz. of additional concentrated protein such as tuna or grilled chicken.

Quinoa salad

* 1 1/2 cups quinoa, rinsed
* two heads radicchio, chopped
* one large English cucumber, cut in quarters
* 1/2 small red onion, diced
* 1 cup cherry or grape tomatoes, halved
* 1 1/2 cups Italian parsley, chopped
* 1 1/2 cups mint leaves, chopped
* 3 Tb. pine nuts
* 1/2 cup olive oil
* 1/4 cup red wine vinegar
* one lemon, juiced
* zest of one lemon
* salt and pepper

* In three cups of water and salt, bring quinoa to a boil, cover, and simmer for about fifteen to twenty minutes until water is absorbed. Let quinoa cool. In

the bottom of a large bowl, whisk together olive oil, vinegar, lemon juice, and salt and pepper. Then add all the rest of the ingredients and combine completely.

➡ APPETIZERS

Endive boats
This is a nice appetizer idea I originally got from a good friend who brought it to one of our gatherings. These are easy to make, absolutely delicious, and will impress your guests.

* four heads of endive (white and/or red), trimmed and leaves separated
* 1 cup goat cheese
* 1/2 cup pomegranate seeds
* 1/2 cup toasted walnuts
* balsamic drizzle

- Fill the wide end of each endive leaf with about two to three teaspoons of goat cheese (depending on the size of the leaves). Top each leaf with walnuts and pomegranate seeds. Lay them out on your serving platter and lightly squeeze balsamic drizzle over the endive boats.

Loaded hummus
This is an excellent dip if you are hosting a get together or bringing an appetizer to a party. You can make it ahead, and it holds up well, so that's always a winner. Of course, this is an easy dish to make and keep in your own fridge for snacking or adding as part of meal during the week.

Base

* 2 cups hummus (store-bought works fine, but homemade hummus is a bonus)

Toppings

* 1 cup cucumber, diced

* 1 cup tomatoes, diced

* 1/2 cup chopped olives

* 1/8 cup red onion, diced

* 1/2 cup crumbled feta

* 2 Tb. each of fresh dill and parsley

* olive oil

* lemon juice

• Spread hummus over bottom of a shallow serving bowl or platter. In a mixing bowl, toss together the toppings and then spread them evenly over the hummus, and drizzle with olive oil and lemon juice.

SOUPS

Minestrone

* one large onion, diced

* one leek sliced

* two carrots, chopped

* two celery ribs, chopped

* five cloves garlic chopped

* two small Yukon gold potatoes, peeled, and diced

* two small zucchini, finely chopped
* one small yellow squash, finely chopped
* three medium tomatoes, peeled and finely chopped
* 1 cup green peas
* one 15oz. can cannellini beans, drained and rinsed
* one 15oz. can red kidney beans, drained and rinsed
* 3 Tb. olive oil
* 6 cups broth (chicken or vegetable)—heated
* 2 Tb. fresh marjoram (2 tsp. dried)
* 1 Tb. fresh thyme (1 tsp. dried)
* 1 Tb. fresh chives
* salt and pepper

Toppings

* pesto
* parmesan cheese

• Heat a large Dutch oven, add olive oil and sauté onion and leek for five minutes, then add the carrots, celery, and garlic for about five minutes. Then add the potatoes. After three minutes, pour in the heated stock and add all of the herbs, salt, and pepper. Cover and bring to a boil, and then reduce to a simmer for ten minutes. Add the zucchini and yellow squash and leave for another five minutes, before adding the tomatoes. Simmer for another ten minutes. Then add the green peas and beans for the final ten minutes. Finally, turn off the heat and let stand for fifteen minutes before serving. Top each serving with one teaspoon of pesto and freshly grated parmesan.

Spicy red lentil coconut soup

* four medium red onions
* six cloves of garlic, chopped
* two Thai small chili peppers, seeded and finely chopped
* two-inch piece of lemongrass, trimmed and inside finely sliced
* 2 cups red lentils
* 1 Tb. ground coriander
* 1 Tb. paprika
* 1/2 tsp. ginger
* 3 cups of coconut milk

Toppings:

* 2 cups fresh cilantro, chopped
* six scallions, chopped
* fresh lime juice

* In a large medium pot or Dutch oven, add onions, garlic, chili, and lemongrass and cook until softened, about five minutes. Then add lentils and ground spices and stir to combine, cooking for about one minute. Then add the coconut milk and seven cups of water. Cover and bring to a boil, then simmer for forty-five minutes. Turn off heat and let stand for fifteen minutes. In serving bowls, top with cilantro, scallions, and fresh lime juice.

➡ PLATTERS

Eating by platters is a favorite way of mine to add diversity to your diet. I prepare all types of platters and use them for entertaining and special occasions, but I also will prepare them as part of a family meal or to leave in the fridge for snacking. Here are some ideas:

* raw vegetable platter—this could be just the standard crudités platter but could be themed, like a platter with the vegetables arranged in the shape of a turkey for Thanksgiving

* fruit platter—for example, tropical, red, and blue berries for July 4th

* Mediterranean salad platter

* charcuterie boards (many options, the key is to feature variety and include some unique ingredients that you don't eat daily)

➡ VEGETABLES

Greek herbed potatoes
This is a favorite dish I serve with a classic Greek salad and chicken souvlaki. It takes a little more time to cook, but it is a crowd pleaser.

* 3 pounds Yukon gold potatoes (chopped into wedges) or fingerlings (chopped in half)

* 3/4 cup broth (chicken or vegetable)

* 3/4 cup olive oil

* two lemons, juiced

* ten garlic cloves, crushed

* 2 Tb. oregano (dried)

* salt and pepper
* fresh Italian parsley and mint

- Preheat oven to 400°F. Combine broth, olive oil, lemon juice, garlic, oregano, salt, and pepper in a small bowl. Place the potatoes in a deep-sided baking dish and pour all of the liquid mixture over the potatoes and toss to combine. Bake uncovered for forty minutes. Turn potatoes and spoon liquid over them to fully coat again. Bake for another thirty to forty minutes until browned. Sprinkle with fresh parsley and mint to serve.

Provençal mushrooms

Some mushrooms like chanterelles can be very expensive and aren't always available. To get more variety in your mushroom in your diet, I suggest using less expensive creminis (which still have excellent health benefits) as the base of the dish and adding in other mushrooms to heighten the complexity of flavor and bioactives in the meal. Of course, the addition of herbs to this dish provides even more diversity.

* 8 oz. cremini mushrooms (thickly slice)
* 4 oz. shiitake mushrooms (thickly slice and discard the stems)
* 4 oz. oyster mushrooms (separate and discard the stems)
* 3 oz. chanterelles (leave small ones whole, half the larger ones)
* 2 Tb. herbes de Provence
* 1 Tb. olive oil
* 1 Tb. grass-fed butter
* salt and pepper

- Melt butter and oil in a sauté pan and add all of the mushrooms to the pan. Sauté for about five minutes, then add herbes de Provence, toss and cook about ten more minutes until the mushrooms are slightly softened and lightly browned. Season with salt and pepper. Optional: plate with a dollop of fresh goat cheese.

Savory sweet Brussels sprouts

This phytonutrient-loaded recipe is my favorite way to prepare Brussels sprouts. Even my husband, who doesn't love Brussels, really enjoys these. The combination of the savory garlic and the bittersweet molasses complements the Brussels perfectly. It's also much quicker than roasting in the oven, getting them to your table faster.

* 1 pound Brussels sprouts

* three cloves garlic, crushed

* 1 Tb. blackstrap molasses

* 1 Tb. olive oil

* 2 Tb. butter

* salt and pepper

1. Trim and cut the Brussels sprouts in half.

2. Add butter and olive oil to a large, heated sauté pan at medium heat until the butter is completely melted.

3. Place Brussels sprouts cut side down in the pan without turning them for about five minutes, until they have a golden and seared appearance on the cut side.

4. Turn all the Brussels sprouts over, leaving a clearing in the center of the pan. Add a small amount of oil before putting the crushed garlic in, cooking it for about thirty seconds.

5. Toss the Brussels sprouts with the garlic.

6. Add two tablespoons of water and then the molasses, stirring to coat.

7. Lower the heat and continue to cook a few more minutes until tender when pierced with a fork.

8. Remove Brussels sprouts from the pan onto a serving dish and enjoy.

Cauliflower mash

A common side dish that goes with almost anything, cauliflower mash is the perfect substitute for mashed potatoes.

* two heads cauliflower
* 3 tablespoons olive oil
* 3/4 cup milk or milk alternative
* 1 teaspoon nutmeg, freshly ground
* three cloves garlic, minced
* 1/2 teaspoon salt
* freshly ground black pepper

• Loosely separate each head of cauliflower into five or six sections and steam until tender. Place cooked cauliflower in food processor with the rest of ingredients until it reaches similar texture to mashed potatoes.

✎ SAUCES

Chimichurri sauce

You can add this classic Argentinian sauce to freshly cooked concentrated protein. I love that this sauce is uncooked and provides a big punch of bioactives.

* 2 cups fresh Italian parsley
* 2/3 cup fresh mint leaves
* 2 Tb. fresh oregano
* one small shallot, diced
* 2 Tb. capers
* three cloves of garlic
* 1 tsp. red pepper flakes
* 2 Tb. red or white wine vinegar
* 2 Tb. lemon juice
* 1/4 tsp. salt and pepper
* 2/3 cup olive oil

* Add all ingredients except olive oil to a food processor and pulse to blend. Scrape down the sides of the bowl and then start blending again while slowly streaming in olive oil until it gets well combined. This sauce can be poured over your protein right before serving.

Other sauces packed with bitter bioactives include:

* Indian curry or tikka masala
* Pesto
* Puttanesca
* Marinara

* Smooth green chutney
* Spicy chili

➡ CONCENTRATED PROTEIN

Greek cod
This is probably my favorite fish dish of all time. It's a big hit with my entire family.

* 2 pounds cod fillet pieces
* eight cloves garlic, crushed
* 1/3 lemon juice
* 1/3 cup olive oil
* 2 Tb. grass-fed butter, melted
* 1/2 cup whole grain flour
* 1 Tb. ground coriander
* 1/2 Tb. ground cumin
* 1/2 Tb. paprika
* 1 tsp. oregano, dried
* Salt and pepper
* fresh parsley, chopped

• Preheat oven to 400°F. You will need two bowls for dipping the cod and a cast iron pan to start it out in before transferring to the oven. In one bowl, combine lemon juice, olive oil, and melted butter. In the second bowl, combine the flour, spices, salt and pepper. First dip the fish in the oil mixture, followed by the spiced flour mixture. Heat a cast iron pan and add three tablespoons of olive oil. Sear fish a few minutes on each side. Drizzle the fillets with the remaining lemon and oil mixture and transfer to the heated oven for about eight to ten minutes. Sprinkle with fresh parsley before serving.

Chicken souvlaki

This is a fun and flavorful way to prepare chicken on skewers. It's great for a family meal, entertaining and makes for great leftover chicken to add to a salad.

* 2 pounds boneless, skinless chicken breasts—cut into medium-sized pieces

* 1/3 cup olive oil

* 3 Tb. lemon juice

* four cloves garlic, crushed

* 2 tsp. oregano, dried

* salt and pepper

• Combine olive oil, lemon juice, garlic, and oregano in the bottom of a baking dish. Add chicken and toss to completely coat. Cover and marinate in the fridge for two to three hours. Skewer the chicken pieces and grill for about fifteen minutes, turning halfway through, until chicken is completely cooked. (You can also skip the skewers and bake in the oven at 400°F for twenty-five to thirty minutes, until chicken is completely cooked.) Serve with tzatziki sauce.

🐛 DESSERTS

Chia seed spice pudding

Although I placed this pudding in the dessert category, I often eat this for breakfast (without the sweetener). This is a supercharged alternative to tapioca pudding. In this version, I use pumpkin pie spices, but you can easily modify it to a classic vanilla or chocolate version. Chia seeds are also a rich source of omega-3s, protein, and fiber.

* 3 cups unsweetened coconut, flax, or almond milk
* 1 cup chia seeds
* 1 tsp. ground spices: cinnamon, cloves, nutmeg etc.
* 1 Tb. agave
* fresh berries

• In a large bowl whisk together milk, chia seeds, agave, and spices. Let sit for at least two hours before serving to allow the chia seeds to plump up. Top with fresh berries to serve.

Pumpkin-coconut flan

Cucurbitacins impart the bitter taste in pumpkin and other squash, including zucchini, summer squash, and melon. This is a great fall and Thanksgiving or special occasion dessert.

* one 15oz. can of pumpkin
* 1 cup canned coconut milk (shake can before opening)
* 2 large eggs
* 1/3 cup agave nectar
* 1 1/2 tsp. cinnamon
* 1/2 tsp. ginger
* 1/2 tsp. nutmeg
* 1/8 tsp. ground cloves
* 1/8 tsp. salt
* 1/4 tsp. vanilla extract

1. Preheat oven to 375°F. Grease a 1 1/2 L(Qt.) baking dish with coconut oil. You will also need a larger dish to place this dish into a water bath (bain-marie) to bake.

2. Mix together all the spices and salt. Beat in the eggs to mix well and then add agave nectar, pumpkin, coconut milk, and vanilla. Combine well until there are no lumps.

3. Transfer to the baking dish and then add water to the larger outer baking dish so the water goes halfway up the side of the dish containing the flan.

4. Bake for about fifty-five minutes until it is set and a toothpick comes out clean.

5. Cool completely before serving. This dish should be served cold.

- Optional: top with whipped cream and pomegranate seeds (another great source of bitters).

CHAPTER 11

Nutritional Supplements

The role of nutritional supplements is to augment the effects of a balanced diet. You can't expect to address the aging process by just taking some supplements if you aren't living the lifestyle, too. While nutritional supplements can provide quick relief from bothersome symptoms or even effective treatment for medical conditions, they cannot undo the body-wide effects of an unhealthy lifestyle. If you are considering adding nutritional supplements to your lifestyle, especially if you take prescription medications or have a medical condition, you should first discuss this with a licensed health care provider knowledgeable about nutrition.

➡ FOUNDATIONAL SUPPORT

When I think about nutritional supplementation for people over thirty-five, I first consider what I refer to as "foundational support." Making sure core macronutrient and micronutrient requirements are being met is my initial goal. In this population, I often recommend three nutritional supplements to provide core support:

* Multivitamin/mineral complex with added bioactives
* Vitamin D
* Omega-3s

The other factor I consider to be foundational is adequate levels of protein and collagen. As we age, we become more susceptible to protein deficiency, mostly because we tend to absorb protein poorly. As I discussed in the first section of the book, improving absorption rates can be addressed through improving digestive health. Oftentimes, I still find many people have trouble getting optimal amounts of protein intake, mostly due to a busy lifestyle, so I may then recommend adding a protein shake to supplement dietary intake of protein.

SUPPLEMENTAL PROTEIN

When choosing a protein powder, it's very important to select protein blends that have a high digestibility score. Because liquid protein passes through the stomach more quickly than a solid meal, you need protein that breaks down easily. If you find that you still have adverse effects (typically gas and/or diarrhea), then you may need a digestive enzyme supplement with protease to help break down the proteins in the shake.

One of my favorite protein sources that plays multiple roles in supporting healthy function is mushroom-fermented plant protein powder. The one I use is sourced from shiitake mushrooms and has added medicinal mushrooms. Not only is it a good source of all of the essential amino acids, but it is highly digestible, making it well suited for the needs of aging. It also contains bitter bioactives which enhance digestive health and other bioactive compounds that support the immune system. Another form of supplemental protein I recommend is sourced from organic yellow peas, and because of its unique composition of branched-chain amino acids and its high digestibility score, it makes a great choice for supporting healthy muscle mass. There's also an organic pea protein with added greens, which is a great way of getting even more of these super foods in your daily diet.

➡ COLLAGEN

In recent years, collagen supplements have become very popular, and I routinely have patients ask me whether or not they should take this supplement. Collagen makes up about 30 percent of the body's total protein, and it's the primary structure of all our connective tissue. The types of collagen we find in our diet are very similar to the main types of collagen in our body. There are sixteen different types of collagen in the body, but the most important types to supplement with that are Types 1, 2, and 3. By just reading the label on a product, you will not usually be able to tell what types of collagen are contained inside, because it will typically just read "collagen peptides." You will have to dig further and likely visit the manufacturer's website to find out where the collagen is sourced from and what types it contains. It's important to take only patented forms of collagen that have scientific clinical evidence to support the product's use in bone and joint health and skin elasticity. It generally takes three to four months to observe noticeable effects on joint and skin health.

➡ TARGETED DIGESTIVE SUPPORT

In the first section of the book, I discussed digestive health extensively. If you are having digestive issues, you should seek the advice of a licensed health care provider and get an accurate diagnosis to help determine if nutritional supplements could be helpful for your condition. Some of the most common supplements I use for digestive support include:

* Digestive enzymes
* Probiotics
* Herbal antimicrobials
* Fiber

* Betaine HCl with pepsin
* Bitter herbs
  * Gentian (*Gentiana lutea*)
  * Dandelion (*Taraxacum officinale*)
  * Lemon balm (*Melissa officinalis*)
  * Fennel (*Foeniculum vulgare*)
  * Ginger (*Zingiber officinale*)

➨ SUPPORT FOR HEALTHY AGING

As I reviewed in the first chapter of this book when I discussed the aging process, reducing oxidative stress and inflammation is very important as you get older. There are so many nutritional supplements that have the ability to act as antioxidants and impact the inflammatory pathway. If you are following the dietary essentials from the Bitter Prescription, then you are getting many of these phytonutrients in your diet already. However, there's also the issue that, as you age, levels of some compounds that we produce in our own body, such as Coenzyme Q10 and GG, tend to decline, and supplementation may provide some benefit. Here are the supplements that I tend to recommend the most:

* Antioxidant phytonutrients/bioactives
  * Blueberry
  * Broccoli
  * Citrus bioflavonoids
  * Curcumin
  * EGCG (green tea extract)
  * "Greens and reds" powders
  * Lycopene

- Quercetin
- Resveratrol

* Coenzyme Q10

* Geranylgeraniol (GG)

* Tocotrienol, delta and gamma (best form of vitamin E)

* Specialized pro-resolving mediators (SPMs)

☛ STRESS AND SLEEP SUPPORT

Managing your body's stress response and getting good quality sleep are essential to your overall health. Chronic stress is a cause of premature aging. In chapter 5, I reviewed the stress response system and the sleep cycle. I also discussed the usefulness of nutritional supplements in supporting the body to have a more balanced response to stressors in our lives and in helping re-establish a more balanced sleep cycle. These are some of the most common supplements I use in my practice:

* Adaptogenic medicinal herbs

- Ashwagandha (*Withania somnifera*)
- Eleuthero (*Eleutherococcus senticosus*)
- Licorice (*Glycyrrhiza glabra*)
- Rhodiola (*Rhodiola rosea*)

* Nutrients for stress support

- Fish oil
- Magnesium
- Phosphatidylserine
- Vitamins B2, B5, and B6
- Vitamin C

* Sleep support

- Chamomile (*Matricaria recutita*)
- GABA
- Lemon balm *(Melissa officinalis)*
- L-theanine
- Magnesium
- Melatonin
- Passionflower (*Passiflora incarnata*)
- Valerian (*Valeriana officinalis*)

ADDRESSING NUTRIENT DEFICIENCIES ASSOCIATED WITH AGING

You should work with a licensed health care provider to determine if you have nutrient deficiencies. Understanding deficiency states can be complex and if supplementation is warranted, it needs to be monitored by your doctor. For example, although iron deficiency can be more common as you get older, it does not mean you should just assume you have it. You should also not start taking iron to prevent an iron deficiency, because iron can be toxic to the liver if levels get too high. Blood tests for iron are widely available. However, low levels of iron may be the result of other medical problems, such as internal bleeding, which is why you need to be under the care of a physician. Also, in some medical conditions and with use of certain medications, supplements may be contraindicated.

Here are the most common deficiencies in people over fifty years old for which supplementation *may* be advised:

* Calcium

* Folate

* Iron

* Magnesium
* Potassium
* Trace minerals
* Vitamin B6
* Vitamin B12
* Vitamin C
* Vitamin D
* Vitamin E

SECTION 3

Executing the Bitter Prescription

CHAPTER 12

Lifestyle Change and Compliance

*W*hat attracted you to this book? How did you come into possession of it? Was it to shed those extra pounds you just can't seem to get rid of? Fix your digestion? Was it because you were diagnosed with a medical condition and you decided it's time to turn your life around and start some new healthy habits or overhaul your diet? Did someone give it to you? Perhaps you heard me in an interview, and something I said struck a chord with you. Did you see me speaking somewhere and wanted to dive deeper into this material? Maybe you heard me reference bitter feelings, and it stirred something in you.

Are you in that category where you've tried every new dietary plan out there only to realize in the end that something was missing? Why didn't those plans work for you? Of course, there is the chance that those plans might not even work for you or produce the results you are looking for. However, often what is missing is the discussion about what keeps us from sticking to a new plan long term. And that is another unique part of the *Bitter Prescription*. This third section of the book reviews how to gain better success in executing this plan in order to get the intended results.

After reading this book, I imagine you going to the grocery store and buying some new types of produce that you've never bought in the past. I imagine you wondering how all this stuff was right in front of you and you never gave it a second glance. I imagine you wondering to yourself how you walked into this same store, picking up the same ingredients over and over again, never taking notice of any of the rest. Well, that is a metaphor for life. Appreciation of your surroundings requires us to be intentional, present, and not feeling bitter. Then, you start to see things in a whole new light. You see things that were there all along and realize you just never noticed them before.

The concepts I am talking about in this book are really quite simple. This is not rocket science. If you have excess fat to lose, I am encouraging you to eat less calories overall. I want you to eat less sugar and processed carbs. You may also need to give your body a bit more of a break from eating, not just the time you spend sleeping, but extend that break into the evening and stop snacking after dinner. I want you to incorporate a greater variety of plants into your diet. I am suggesting you might benefit from taking some supplements to meet your changing digestive and metabolic needs, as you get older.

All of these seemingly simple suggestions have one thing in common. They all involve making a change in your life, and change can be uncomfortable. You have to be in the right state of mind to make any change in your life. I know this, because I have worked with thousands of patients, and if they are not in a good place emotionally, lifestyle changes are very challenging. Okay, maybe they can get started and stick it out for a few weeks, but it is very likely not to last. Furthermore, the concepts in this book are not a quick fix, not a ten- or thirty-day plan. The core principles of the *Bitter Prescription* are intended to help you get and stay healthy for a lifetime. You would never believe that, by completing just a ten-day exercise program, you could radically shift the state of your health for the long run. You know that in order to reap the benefits of exercise, you need to stick to it. It needs to be a regular part of your lifestyle. Simply put, this is the same mindset you need to apply to your dietary habits. It comes down to one word, compliance.

⊷ COMPLIANCE

In my clinical practice, it became apparent pretty quickly that starting patients on a solid lifestyle plan was the easy part. The more difficult part of practicing lifestyle medicine is figuring out how to keep people on track. I would routinely hear from my patients that, even though they experienced great results and felt amazing when they first committed to eating well and staying physically active, that they had so much trouble getting back on track when they were derailed by some issue or stressor that surfaced in their lives. It also became clear that a common thread was a change in their emotional health, often described to me as being thrown into a rut and not being able to get back out. At that point, just reviewing the original dietary plan was clearly not enough to motivate them to move back toward the healthy lifestyle changes they had been successful with initially.

The term in the medical community for when a patient follows the treatment plan, whether it's prescription medicines or lifestyle change, is compliance. This compliance issue, I would discover, would be at the core of what I would encounter with almost every patient. At first, I couldn't understand why someone would just stop following a plan that made them feel so much better. In some of these early cases, this would even occur in people who had amazing results, having lost fifty pounds, being able to get off their blood pressure medication and even seeing their cholesterol and blood sugar levels getting back to normal. But, here we would sit, many months later, and they would explain to me how bad they felt that they had reverted back to their old habits and the weight had come back on, and we would find that their blood test results were back to where they had been. And I continued to wonder why. Why was this happening to so many people?

As I had shared earlier, I had always had a thirst for knowledge and collected information from a young age. Now, the collection became focused on human behavior and what makes someone successful. Luckily, there is a tremendous body of literature to access, especially in the area of career and financial success, which I realized could be applied to healthy lifestyle changes as well. As I continued to work with my patients and apply what I was learning from my study of human behavior, I was able to connect the dots and bridge some of the gaps I was experiencing in my clinical practice. Over the course of many years, I discovered that the patients who were more successful with compliance tended to have a more positive mindset. Furthermore, those who had a positive mindset tended to have fewer bitter feelings.

➡ MIND-BODY CONNECTION

Now, I don't want you thinking that having a positive mindset and peaceful emotional state is only for the purpose of making healthy lifestyle choices. Maintaining a great state of mental health is a key pillar of vitality. We know that depression is an independent risk factor for cardiovascular disease and not simply because depression is causing the person to make poor lifestyle choices. A healthy mind is just as important as a healthy body. Mind and body are inseparable. The health of the body impacts the health of the mind and vice versa.

What follows in this third section of the book is, first, an exploration of what I refer to as bitter thoughts and feelings which are literally toxic to our health. I also discuss how to overcome these bitter feelings. Once these bitter feelings are addressed, then we are in a better state of emotional health to start working on our mindset. And, finally, when we shift to a more positive mindset, we are in the best place to work on our daily habits, which make up our lifestyle and affect our overall health, and keep us feeling on track and, most importantly, balanced.

CHAPTER 13

Bitter Feelings

*L*et me start out by making a clear distinction regarding mental health. In my medical practice, I routinely treat patients who are suffering from very clinically significant mood and cognitive disorders. People with symptoms of depression, anxiety, post-traumatic stress disorder, and/or bipolar disorder (and the list goes on) should seek care from a licensed and trained medical professional. Just being told that you should change your thought patterns and become happier and less irritable is far from an effective treatment.

There is so much hope now for improving and balancing your mental health, especially with using integrative medicine, that incorporates not just the standard approach of medication and psychotherapy, but also takes the form of whole-body medicine, including modalities like acupuncture, neurotherapy, meditation, yoga, light therapy, breath work, spirituality, herbal medicine, and, of course, nutrition and dietary therapy. It is very important to develop a trusted relationship with your health care provider, one that provides a state where you feel educated and empowered about your overall health. Very often, this is the focus of the work I do with patients. I view mental health as a core element of your overall health, and at any point in time, we sit somewhere along the spectrum. Addressing bitter thoughts and feelings in the context of a mental health condition can be part of the treatment plan, but just this alone is not enough. So please make sure you are taking the steps you need, which may include working with a mental health professional.

⬤ BITTER THOUGHTS AND FEELINGS

I hope you are ready, because this is where we need to start talking about the uncomfortable stuff. The "I'm a failure again," the "I'm emotionally exhausted," the "I'm not good enough" self-dialogue that runs through our heads. While this is not true for everyone, I have seen many times that a fundamental belief in lack of worthiness, lack of self-love, and neglecting self-care can lead to numbing emotion through food. As I mentioned in the first section of the book, there are specific genes that can result in people being more likely to demonstrate the behavior of an "emotional eater." In that case, when a person is under stress, they can be more likely to turn to food for comfort. I also reviewed that even the bacteria that reside in your gut can communicate with your brain, actually changing your emotions to influence your eating behavior, which may also need to be addressed.

Here, I want to talk more about the bitter thoughts that can keep a running dialogue, creeping up on us as we get in bed, as we wake up at night, as we drive our kids around from soccer practice to piano lessons, which may go like this:

"I am secretly afraid that I am going to melt down and no longer be able to keep up with the demands of my life. I am tired. I am stressed. I am trying too hard and barely getting by, never getting ahead. If I step up in one area, then things fall apart in another. I don't have enough time to do it all. I want to contribute more, be a better mother and wife, be more present, be better at work, but I don't have the energy or will to do it anymore. Sometimes I feel like I am wishing away time so I can finally get a break, but I am afraid that when that break comes, I will have wished away the best years of my life. I worry about failure. I worry about our finances. I worry about my health and my family's health. My biggest fear is that I worry that I am the engine that

keeps all this going, and if I slow down or stop, it will all come crashing down. No one else can do everything that I do. I don't have anyone to rely on and to back me up. I don't face the future, because I am uncertain of my abilities to perform and to get to where I used to dream of being. I worry about disappointing people, about not being good enough. Other people think I have it all together and that I am an amazing success, but I never feel like I measure up to that. I am afraid I have to do more and more to show that I am a success. And then, I am also afraid that I don't know if I am on the right path. Am I here doing what I am supposed to be doing? I don't feel like I have the time, the mindset, or am in the right mood to figure it out. I wish people around me understood how demanding life really is for me and how little time I have. I secretly wish that I could have it all. I really do want to have unlimited time and the emotional presence to enjoy life. I want to experience a joyful family life and feel a purpose-fulfilled life. But I just don't know where to start."

Can you identify with this? This is how many people really feel right now. They may not say all of this in this much detail to you, but these are the types of thoughts that keep many of your friends up at night. This is an all-too-common presence I encounter in both my professional and personal life. In fact, there have been times when I have felt this way. I believe it is time we really get this out in the open, break it down, and address it piece by piece, because it is literally destroying people, families, and communities. There is such a crisis of mental health and chronic disease today, and we need to turn this around. These two topics are often discussed separately, but the mind and body are so deeply connected that there really is no separation, and in order to effectively make change, both must be addressed.

The state of your emotional health matters and affects the aging process at least equally to dietary habits, if not more. Bitter thoughts and feelings, like blame and resentment, stress, irritability, anger, and pessimism, can sabotage your health. Essentially, bitter thoughts create these bitter feelings which are perceived by the body as emotional stress, and, left unchecked, these emotions ultimately impact how your genes get expressed. Simply put, stressful and negative thought patterns can impact the body at the DNA level and affect overall health.

Examples of bitter thoughts

* I can't get anyone to help me with this, so I have to do it all on my own.

* I have my parents to blame for this.

* Most of my co-workers annoy me.

* Why is everyone else getting ahead at work instead of me?

* I can't stand my boss.

* I will never get ahead.

* I am stuck in a dead-end job or relationship.

* My spouse/partner should help out more.

* It's all their fault that I am stressed out like this.

* Things won't get any better than this.

Rumination, where the thoughts play over and over again like a recording, adds more power to these thoughts, which then causes the experience of feeling the bitter emotions. Let's put a name to these bitter feelings:

* Agitation

* Anger

* Blame
* Envy
* Fear
* Guilt
* Greed
* Indifference
* Irritation
* Resentment
* Shame
* Stress
* Worry

It is beyond the scope of this book to address in any depth all of these feelings, and I can't even begin to come close to the level of expertise of some amazing people in the field of emotional health, like Brené Brown and her work on shame. I would encourage you to explore this area more as there are entire books devoted to these topics. So, let me briefly take you through my take on a couple of the most common bitter feelings affecting us.

Blame and resentment
Bitterness can take the form of blame and resentment. You may feel your life circumstances are someone else's fault. You may blame your negative feelings on your spouse or your sister or your boss. Of course, events may occur, or have occurred, in your life that are the result of someone else's wrongdoing and are certainly not your fault. What I am referring to here is your reaction to these events and the feeling of not having control over your own emotional state. Any psychotherapist can tell you that continually living with a sense of blame against

someone who wronged you in the past does much more harm to your health than it does to the person you are directing the bitter feeling against. Once you are able to break free from blame and instead embrace the empowering mode of taking responsibility for how you feel and how your life is going, you will feel a huge shift in your emotional state.

Irritation and stress

Feeling irritable and overreacting to situations are the main complaints that my patients describe to me. They tell me they are snapping at their kids and spouse. They can't let go of little things that they say shouldn't bother them as much as they do. They go to bed thinking about what went wrong during the day and have trouble falling asleep, as they replay the events of the day. They wake up at night thinking about what they need to do the next day, the problems they have to face. They describe blowing things out of proportion in the middle of the night and having difficulty getting back to sleep. They know they don't like the way they feel but don't know how to get out of the cycle.

How stress and worry can become habits that make you unhappy

Not unlike other addictions, people can become stuck in the vicious cycle of "rewarding" themselves with more unhappiness when they practice the mindless, habitual activities and thought patterns that lead them to wishing time away. When you get up feeling the burden of the day that lies ahead of you, running a preview tape of everything you need to do that day, it should come as no surprise that you will wish the day was over before it even begins and look forward to getting back into the bed you just got up from.

Some of the worst habits I see in my patients are not getting enough sleep, too much stress that is not managed well, and not enough exercise. Then, people can be more likely to fall into the trap of making poor food choices, either because they are stressed or because of the sense of too little time to plan meals. It's a widespread issue. We are spread way too thin and have trouble finding our way back to balance until something serious starts happening with our health that often sends us to the doctor's office.

Unhappiness habits

It is important to name and define as many unhappiness habits as possible that may be present in your life so that you can begin to identify how much this is consuming and destroying your life. There are four main unhappiness habits that I see in my practice that are affecting the overall sense of well-being of my patients.

1. Social media

    *   How do you typically feel after spending an extended period of time scrolling your feed? This habit often doesn't make people feel happier and better about themselves or their life in general. Mainly, people feel defeated, resentful, jealous...bitter about life and how they don't measure up to all of those high points of life that they see posted on social media. Yet, they continue to go right back on there, often many times daily.

2. Disconnected from nature

    *   The simple act of spending more time outside, immersed in nature, can reduce the perception of stress and improve emotional health. Studies have even shown that residents in urban areas who are exposed to more trees experience less

anxiety. When people spend more time outside moving around in their green surroundings (what I like to call "green light therapy") they display reductions in physical signs of stress such as muscle tension and pulse rate.

3. Poor relationships

*   When you ask people what matters most to them, they will often cite their loved ones. Maintaining healthy relationship takes both intention and time. Because many people feel so overwhelmed and have a sense of not having enough time in the day to get everything done, they will often drop spending quality time with their family and friends. Also, if they are distracted and not feeling present during those interactions, relationships can suffer.

SOCIAL CONNECTION

A surprising predictor of poor health is lack of social connection. Maintaining meaningful relationships can increase survival by 50 percent. Being disconnected from others, having few social connections has been shown to be a risky health behavior and is:

*   Equivalent to being an alcoholic or smoking fifteen cigarettes per day
*   Worse than not exercising
*   Twice as harmful as obesity!

SELF-CRITICISM

At the root of self-criticism is a poor sense of self-worth, lack of self-love, and ultimately, shame. More than half of women harbor negative thoughts about themselves weekly. This is a deep-rooted issue that is worsened by stress, making people in our fast-paced society much more vulnerable to negative self-judgement.

Aging, unhappiness, and the *U* curve

According to the *U*-curve theory, people are at their most unhappy in their forties, and once they reach their fifties, happiness begins to return. Unfortunately, the forties are a very sensitive time when the lifestyle choices we make can seriously impact our long-term health. If we feel emotionally drained and unhappy, it makes it even harder to put the effort into creating health instead of chronic disease.

Clearing bitter feelings

For a small minority, getting rid of bitter feelings can be as simple as figuring out what really makes you happy and putting more of that into your daily life. But for most of us, that method doesn't work and requires a deeper commitment to working on yourself. So it comes as no surprise that the self-help section in libraries and bookstores is extensive. Meditation is one of the core practices I would recommend to everyone, because as I mentioned in section one, it helps rewire the pathways in the brain that are involved in fear and promotes a state of calmness. Here are three more daily practices to help reframe your thought patterns, flip that switch, and change how you are perceiving your world:

1. Taking charge

What I am referring to here is accepting responsibility for your thoughts. Only you can change your thought patterns. Of course, this can take some hefty self-work, potentially with a trained psychotherapist. By accepting responsibility for your own pattern of thoughts, you can keep the bitter feelings of resentment and blame in check.

Stop being so hard on yourself! At any given moment, we should only expect ourselves to show up as the best version of our self in that unique set of circumstances. What derails us is expecting that there is some pedestal we must sit on all the time, no matter what the setting. If you were acutely ill with the flu, you wouldn't expect to be setting a personal record on your one-mile run. In fact, you really wouldn't expect much of yourself at all, and would accept the current situation as it is, and give yourself a break, and hopefully rest to recover. Here are some other ways to help take charge of how your feelings:

* Make a pledge to stop complaining
* Make another pledge to stop gossiping
* Stop holding grudges and work on forgiveness (this can be one of the most profound shifts that you can make to affect your emotional health)

2. Practicing gratitude

The practice of gratitude is one of the best methods to change the pattern of your thoughts that influence your emotional health. When you are grateful for your life as it is currently, it becomes much harder to feel bitter feelings towards others and yourself. Research is actually showing that people who practice gratitude are less likely to feel anxious or depressed.

Count your blessings

Simply start by making a list of things, people, or experiences in your life for which you are grateful. I typically recommend getting a notebook, noting the date at the top, and writing down at least three new things (that you haven't listed recently) that make you feel blessed. If you can write a list of ten, even better. It is also important to evoke the feelings of gratitude while you are writing. The longer you are in this state, the better. Recording your blessings in the morning is a great way to start the day.

Evening reflection

This is a simple technique I developed and advise to my patients. Before going to sleep, close your eyes and reflect back on your day and think of the instances when you felt your best, when you felt a sense of peace, purpose, or love in your life. Try to come up with five of these, and you will often find these were very simple moments during the day.

Grace

Before you eat anything, state how thankful you are for the food your body is about to receive. This does not need to be religious, although if you are already in the habit of saying grace as a religious practice, that is wonderful, but take a moment to make sure you are truly evoking the emotions of gratitude. This calms your system, which is very important for eating. You need your parasympathetic nervous system active for proper digestion. The very thought of food also primes your system to switch to digest mode.

3. Staying present and feeling connected
Staying present and aware of signs of connection and all the goodness that arrives into your life daily is a wonderful way to help rewire thought patterns and restore a sense of

inner balance. This requires becoming more mindful of the present moment, and there are a few ways to help better promote this state, including time segmentation, creativity, and service.

Time segmentation

An excellent way I have found to feel more present and limit distracting thoughts is through the practice of time segmentation. This means that you think about your day as a series of small activities. You make a statement to yourself that one activity is ending and the next is beginning. While you are in that activity, such as driving to work, you stay focused on that and make a pledge to not think ahead to other parts of the day or think back to the past.

Creativity

The process of creation puts us in the zone where we can feel our own strength. It also makes us feel present. When you are creative, you are in a powerful energetic and emotional state. People overestimate what creativity really means. When I talk to patients about being creative, I often get responses like "I'm just not a creative person" or "I don't have time to do anything creative." But being a creative person exhibits many different appearances. Creation is not reserved for professional artists. It is for every single one of us. Creativity can be complex at times, but it is mostly simplistic acts. Creativity can be the way you lay out food on your plate. It can be organizing your desk drawer or planting flowers near your front door. When you use your creative muscle, you are also rewiring your brain and emotions to be in a state of happiness.

Service

Opportunities abound to help people in need. If you already routinely volunteer your time for a cause, then you know how good it makes you feel. Random acts of kindness on a regular basis can have the same effect. Service to others helps you get outside of yourself. Perhaps you offer to take another person's shopping cart back from the parking lot, or you drop a few extra items into the food donation bin at the grocery store. When you consistently ask yourself, "How can I be of service today?" without expecting anything in return, then you are in service for the greater good. I believe helping is a natural tendency and leads to a deeper sense of connection, not only within our communities but on a grander scale. While I think that service to others is what matters most in life, there are also physical benefits from helping behaviors. A recent study of more than four thousand people with heart disease demonstrated that, those who spent time providing non-paid assistance to family and friends outside of their households, experienced fewer depressive symptoms compared to those who provided no assistance. Those in the "helping" group also decreased their chances of having another cardiac event or dying in the two years in which they were followed.

➡ BITTER FEELINGS AND FOOD

Most of this chapter has been devoted to overall emotional health which, as I stated, is critical to your physical health. There are also feelings directly related to food preparation and eating habits that can impact your emotional state.

Food fretting

Food fretting is a behavior that can also be viewed as "food stress," and it can impact your feelings. Here, I am referring to the actual process of selecting what to eat, and for some people, this can be quite stressful. This is a modern-day issue created from the bombardment of differing messages about what is healthy and unhealthy to eat and can come from many sources, including the nutrition industry, government, advertisers, the media, and even lobbyists. There are so many voices in the field now that even a health care provider trained in nutrition can have difficulty knowing who to trust for reliable advice.

Preparing food with love

When I first came across the following esoteric quote, I was struck most by the last sentence that references preparing food while experiencing bitter feelings. Have you experienced food prepared in the setting of love and how much better you feel enjoying that meal? No doubt, if you are in a good mood while making a meal and enjoying the experience of sharing a meal with others, you will feel better.

"If a woman could see the sparks of light going forth from her fingertips when she is cooking, and the substance of light that goes into the food she handles, she would be amazed to see how much of herself she charges into the meals that she prepares for her family and friends. It is one of the most important and least understood activities of life, that the radiation and feeling that go into the preparation of food affect everyone who partakes of it. And this activity should be unhurried, peaceful, and happy because the substance of the lifestream performing the service flows into that food and is eaten, and actually becomes part of the energy of the receiver. It would be better that an individual did not eat at all than to eat food that has been prepared under a feeling of anger, apathy, resentment, depression, or any outward pressure."—Maha Chohan, *Electrons*

➥ SETTING EMOTIONAL HEALTH CHECKPOINTS

Similar to how I suggested setting checkpoints for maintaining a healthy body composition, you may want to consider setting emotional health checkpoints to help you maintain your emotional health. Some examples of areas to set defined goals for yourself include:

* Family and social time
* Meditation time
* Service
* Spiritual practice

CHAPTER 14

Positive Mindset

By now, it should be clear that I am a proponent of long-term lifestyle changes as opposed to a quick fix or program. As I stated, the problem is that most people can't commit to long-term change, and this is why many people feel like they aren't succeeding at life. This is why diets can fail. This is why there are free trial gym memberships and unlimited visits, because people stop using them. When you visit the gym in January, it's packed, but come February, it's back to just the regulars. This is why many success experts now correctly label New Year's resolutions as a recipe for failure. And this is why I wrote this third section in this book.

So why is it so difficult to stick to a plan? For many, it can come down to the fact that the discipline it takes is boring for most people. We live in the era of the quick fix, the "take a pill for that," the ten-day master plan. Small mundane changes that produce big results over time don't get many people excited. The promise to get a flat tummy in ten days grabs attention and revs people up, and they jump on the bandwagon. And when they don't end up with the results they were promised, they just go back to their old ways until some other new "program" captures their attention.

The effects of successful habits in any area of life (including relationships, business, finances, and career) are gradual, and in the moment, might be hard to distinguish from failure. For the most part, the same is true of unhealthy habits. Of course, there are exceptions to that rule. However, you gain weight *over time*. Your cells and metabolism change *over time*. And you don't become a type 2 diabetic overnight.

Your lifestyle habits are influenced by your mindset, which influences virtually everything you do. There is an entire self-help industry devoted to the concept of developing a positive attitude. It goes all the way back to Norman Vincent Peale, who wrote *The Power of Positive Thinking* in 1952. He is hailed by many as the father of positive thinking and was one of the most widely read inspirational writers of all time. He said, "There is a real magic in enthusiasm. It spells the difference between mediocrity and accomplishment."

I believe enthusiasm is the hallmark of a robust positive attitude. You will find that people who consider themselves to be optimists are more likely to display enthusiasm in most areas of their lives. There is an entire body of research devoted to studying the health outcomes of people who are considered optimists versus those who are pessimists.

THE HEALING POWER OF HOPE

When it comes down to basics, optimists can find solutions where pessimists cannot. They essentially hold *hope* that there is a better outcome, that things can get better, that the situation can improve. And this is what having a positive mindset is all about.

The research paints a pattern of reduced risk of various diseases in people who have hope, and when they do fall ill, they have better outcomes. Hope can positively affect endorphin release and perception of pain. People who are hopeful practice healthier lifestyle habits, such as vegetable intake, smoking status, safer sex, and exercise.

In research settings, hope is defined in two ways: (1) optimism and (2) a combination of positive belief and expectation. Both of these topics have been the subject of many studies in relation to various health outcomes. Studies often compare people in varying categories on a continuum between optimism and pessimism. Subjects in the highest category of optimism (who would be the most hopeful subjects) have the best cardiovascular health in terms of risk factors from diet, activity level, body mass index, smoker status, blood sugar, and total cholesterol levels. People who are optimistic will fare better after a bypass surgery, reducing their risk of having a heart attack or needing additional procedures or hospitalization by half. On the other hand, pessimists are at higher risk of having a heart attack. Optimists also have a lower risk of developing dementia.

➥ LIFE-VIEW AND PURPOSE

There are quite a few research studies looking at the concept of life-view and the role it plays in health status. Life-view is defined as having broader lifelong goals that serve to direct and organize your day-to-day activities and what you value as having importance in your life. In simple terms, it's the reason why you get up every day and do what you do. It may be that caring for your family is what guides you, or improving the lives of others in a more "professional" setting, or perhaps both. Whatever it is for you, it remains with you throughout the day. And it doesn't have to be complicated. You don't need to enroll in a twelve-month program to find your "true" purpose in life. As I have said, it's as easy as simply doing what ultimately brings you joy. You will feel a sense of peace and flow when you are doing what you love.

Your attitude toward life, whether you generally think things tend to work out or the world is just out to get you, is also key to your well-being. In fact, a recent study showed that cynics end up having a threefold greater risk of developing Alzheimer's and dementia. Optimists, on the other hand, have been observed to have increased longevity. They tend to be more likely to exercise, experience lower levels of stress hormones, and generally take better care of themselves.

Characteristics of people ninety-five years and older include being optimistic, more outgoing, and, in general, easygoing. They also say that laughter is important to them, and they tend to have larger social networks.

☞ THE MULTITASKING MYTH

For many, the ability to multitask is a badge of honor. It's a common addition to the list of proficiencies when applying for a new job. It supposedly separates the highly effective producers from the rest of the pack. But is it really a competitive advantage, and does it lead to greater productivity? And even more importantly, what does it do to our emotional health and mindset? It turns out that multitasking and success do not go hand in hand. We now know that it is quite the opposite. Productivity is actually improved when people focus on one task at a time. This information has even made headlines in recent years, prompting many people to shy away from promoting themselves as a "proficient multitasker." Staying focused on the task at hand can help with staying in a more positive mindset.

☞ WAYS TO SUPPORT A POSITIVE MINDSET

There are many specific ways to help promote the thinking patterns that contribute to a positive mindset. It's very important to make sure reactivity to stressors is being addressed, with meditation being one of the most effective ways to help.

Stress reduction techniques
There are a multitude of techniques that can help better manage stress. Here are some ways to reduce the effects of emotional stress that can affect your mental health and, in turn, your mindset:

* Alternate nostril breathing

* Art and creativity

* Energy work

* Exercise

* Gardening

* Grounding

* Guided imagery

* Meditation

* Progressive relaxation

* Relaxation breathing

* Spending time in nature

* Tai-chi

* Yoga

Reading
There are countless books in the success and positive attitude category that can help with supporting your goal of developing a more positive mindset. As a lifelong learner, I am always reading books about motivation, human behavior, and success. There are so many talented authors in this field with different takes and styles that you should have no trouble finding books that are a good fit for you. Consider committing to reading a minimum of ten pages per day from inspiring books.

Daily awareness technique
Select a nice journal to carry with you and write down instances that show you how wonderful the world is around you in your current life experience. If you are in a rut or feel like nothing is going right in your life, you might say there is nothing to write, but just start by noting the little things, everything from

finding a penny on the floor to someone holding the door open for you. By focusing on the positive things in your life, in effect, you can reduce your stress response by limiting how much time you spend in a state of bitter feelings. This also mimics the view of optimists in that they tend to look on the bright side of things and are looking for the silver lining.

Evening reflection

You may have heard the old saying, "When you are on your death bed and look back at your life, you will see that it was only the small things that mattered." The evening reflection method I developed (discussed in the previous chapter) is an effective tool, and a good starting point to explore what all those "small things" are and, over time, push more of those into our days. This ends up making the stressors in our life seem less significant, and over time, there can be a mindset change to the things that really matter in our lives. Instead of being in a mindset of combating stress, a shift of focus to bringing more joy into our lives is a more effective way to ease tension. By tipping this balance, the body receives more positive biochemical signals. Like anything else, this requires consistency. Changing thought patterns and mental habits that contribute to mindset can take months of dedicated, daily devotion.

Affirmations

Many success experts tout the practice of affirmations as an effective way to promote a positive mindset. They say that in the beginning you may not even fully believe the statements you have prepared, but with repetition and the evocation of positive emotion, over time, these recitations become your positive thoughts. Stating these declarations in front of a mirror may amplify their effect.

Examples of positive affirmations for healthy living:

* "I am becoming happier and healthier every day"

* "I only eat foods that fuel my brain and body for success"

* "I love how eating healthy gives me more energy and makes me feel happier"

* "I feel and look more vibrant every day"

* "I am becoming the best version of myself"

* "I am proud of myself for the healthy choices I make"

* "I love how I feel when I take better care of myself"

* "My life is better when I am committed to caring for myself"

* "I am blessed with wonderful health"

My personal message to you

At the deepest level, when I think about my fundamental belief that fuels my desire to help people, it ultimately comes down to creating a better world for all of us, one person at a time. I believe we all have unique gifts to share here on this earth, and when we feel our best, then we can pour our innate talents and abilities into our life's work and really give it our all.

No matter what your role or profession, whether you are a parent, an entrepreneur, a health care provider, a teacher, an artist, an athlete, an entertainer, an insurance agent, a realtor, or a care-giver for aging parents, when you are feel your best, those around you benefit, and there is no end to how far that goes out into the world, one person at a time, sort of like a ripple effect. My goal is to help you feel your personal best so that you can share who you really are inside. When you feel well—physically, emotionally, and spiritually—the whole world is better for it!